Ancient Babylonian Medicine

Ancient Cultures

These enjoyable, straightforward surveys of key themes in ancient culture are ideal for anyone new to the study of the ancient world. Each book reveals the excitement of discovering the diverse lifestyles, ideals, and beliefs of ancient peoples.

Published

Ancient Babylonian Medicine
Markham J. Geller

The Spartans
Nigel Kennell

Sport and Spectacle in the Ancient World
Donald G. Kyle

Food in the Ancient World
John M. Wilkins and Shaun Hill

Greek Political Thought
Ryan K. Balot

Sexuality in Greek and Roman Culture
Marilyn B. Skinner

Theories of Mythology
Eric Csapo

In preparation

Science in the Ancient World
Daryn Lehoux

Ethnicity and Identity in the Ancient World
Kathryn Lomas

Roman Law and Society
Thomas McGinn

Economies of the Greek and Roman World
Jeremy Paterson

Economies of the Greco-Roman World
Gary Reger

The City of Rome
John Patterson

Family in Greek and Roman Culture
Emma Griffiths and Tim Parkin

Markham J. Geller

Ancient Babylonian Medicine

Theory and Practice

WILEY-BLACKWELL
A John Wiley & Sons, Ltd., Publication

Blackwell Publishing was acquired by John Wiley & Sons in February 2007. Blackwell's publishing program has been merged with Wiley's global Scientific, Technical, and Medical business to form Wiley-Blackwell.

Registered Office
John Wiley & Sons Ltd, The Atrium, Southern Gate, Chichester, West Sussex, PO19 8SQ, United Kingdom

Editorial Offices
350 Main Street, Malden, MA 02148-5020, USA
9600 Garsington Road, Oxford, OX4 2DQ, UK
The Atrium, Southern Gate, Chichester, West Sussex, PO19 8SQ, UK

For details of our global editorial offices, for customer services, and for information about how to apply for permission to reuse the copyright material in this book please see our website at www.wiley.com/wiley-blackwell.

Library of Congress Cataloging-in-Publication Data

Geller, Markham J.
Ancient Babylonian medicine : theory and practice / Markham J. Geller.
v. cm. – (Ancient cultures)
Includes bibliographical references and index.
Contents: Introduction to Babylonian medicine and magic – Medicine as science – Who did what to whom? – The politics of medicine – Medicine as literature – Medicine and philosophy – Medical training : MD or PhD? – Uruk medical commentaries – Medicine and magic as independent approaches to healing – Appendix: An edition of a medical commentary.
ISBN 978-1-119-02552-8 1. Medicine, Assyro-Babylonian.
2. Medicine, Assyro-Babylonian–Philosophy. 3. Medicine, Assyro-Babylonian–Methodology. 4. Magic, Assyro-Babylonian. I. Title.
R135.3.G44 2010
610.938–dc22

2009046375

A catalogue record for this book is available from the British Library.

Set in 10/12.5pt Rotation by SPi Publisher Services, Pondicherry, India

I 2015

To Florentina

Contents

Illustrations

Map

Figures

Abbreviations

AIPHOS	*Annuaire de l'Institut de Philologie et d'Histoire Oriéntales et Slaves* (Brussels)
AMT	R. Campbell Thompson *Assyrian Medical Texts* (London, 1923)
ARM	Archives royales de Mari
ArOr	Archiv Orientální
AuOr	*Aula Orientalis*
BAK	H. Hunger, *Babylonische und assyrische Kolophone* (Neukirchen-Vluyn, 1968)
BAM	F. Köcher, *Babylonisch-assyrische Medizin in Texten und Untersuchungen*, 1–7 (for 7 see Geller 2005)
BE	Babylonian Expedition (BE 17/1 = H. Radau, *Letters to Cassite Kings from the Temple Archives of Nippur* [Philadelphia, 1908])
BRM	Babylonian Records in the Library of J. Pierpont Morgan (see Clay 1923)
BSOAS	*Bulletin of the School of Oriental and African Studies*
CAD	*Chicago Assyrian Dictionary*
CBQ	*Catholic Biblical Quarterly*
CH	Codex Hammurabi
CH E	Codex Hammurabi Epilogue
CRRAI	*Compte Rendu, Rencontre Assyriologique Internationale*
JCS	*Journal of Cuneiform Studies*
JESHO	*Journal of the Economic and Social History of the Orient*
JMC	*Journal des Médecines Cunéiformes*
JANES	*Journal of the Near East Society of Columbia University*
JNES	*Journal of Near Eastern Studies*

JEOL	*Jaarbericht ex Oriente Lux*
JRAS	*Journal of the Royal Asiatic Society*
KAR	*Keilschrifttexte aus Assur religiösen Inhalts*
LKA	*Literarische Keilschrifttexte aus Assur*
MAOG	*Mitteilungen der Altorientalischen Gesellschaft*
MLC	Tablets belonging to the Pierpont Morgan Library (now in the Yale University Babylonian Collection)
MSL	Materials for the Sumerian Lexicon (Rome)
Or	*Orientalia*
RA	*Revue d'assyriologie*
SAA	State Archives of Assyria (see Parpola 1993)
SBTU	Spätbabylonische Texte aus Uruk
STT	*The Sultantepe Tablets*, ed. O. Gurney, J. J. Finkelstein, P. Hulin (London)
TCL	Textes cunéiformes du Louvre (see Thureau-Dangin 1922)
TDP	See Labat 1951
Ut. Lem.	*Utukkū Lemnūtu* incantations (see Geller 2007c)
WZKM	*Wiener Zeitschrift für die Kunde des Morgenlandes*
ZA	*Zeitschrift für Assyriologie*

Acknowledgments

This book was made possible by a grant from the Wellcome Trust, which allowed me to spend the 2005–6 academic year at the Collège de France and École Pratique des Hautes Études, Paris, through the invitation of J.-M. Durand. Further work on the manuscript was carried out during two research visits to the Max Planck Institut für Wissenschaftsgeschichte, Berlin, courtesy of Peter Damerow and Jürgen Renn. These visits were funded by grants from the Alexander von Humboldt-Stiftung (Wiederaufnahme Stipendium) and the TOPOI Excellence Cluster of the Freie Universität Berlin, with Eva Cancik-Kirschbaum as my *Betreurerin.*

The manuscript received a thorough and highly critical reading from Irving Finkel, which resulted in a major redrafting of the text.

I would like to thank a number of colleagues who have generously helped in providing illustrations for this volume. Frans Wiggermann and Dominique Collon kindly sent along their original drawings as well as photos from their own archives, and Tessa Rickards provided her drawing of an object in the Vorderasiatisches Museum, Berlin. Ulla Kasten supplied an old photo from the Yale Babylonian Collection taken by A. T. Clay, with permission to publish it. Béatrice André-Salvini graciously granted permission to publish photos from the Louvre taken by Florentina Badalanova Geller, to whom this volume is dedicated.

Finally, I would like to thank Galen Smith of Wiley-Blackwell for seeing this work through to publication and Clare Creffield for copy-editing the manuscript.

Introduction to Babylonian Medicine and Magic

> If a man has pain in his kidney, his groin constantly hurts him, and his urine is white like donkey-urine, and later on his urine shows blood, that man suffers from "discharge" (*muṣû*-disease). You boil 2 shekels of myrrh, 2 shekels of *baluhhu*-resin, (and) 2 *sila*-measures of vinegar together in a jug; cool it and mix it in equal measure in pressed oil. You pour half into his urethra via a copper tube, half mix in premium beer, you leave it out overnight and he drinks it on an empty stomach and he will get better.
>
> Babylonian recipe for disease of the kidneys, *BAM* 7 35

> [If a] man has intestinal colic, he constantly scratches himself, he retains wind in his anus, food and fluids are regurgitated (and) he suffers from constipation of the rectum – its "redness" is *raised* and troubles him [without] giving him relief – you desiccate a lion skin and mix it with lion fat, you dry (it) a second time, crush and mix it in cedar oil, make a pessary and insert it into his anus.
>
> Babylonian recipe for disease of the anus, *BAM* 7 151

Medicine today is technological and scientific, often making it difficult to cast our minds back to earlier ages when medicine was less understood and less successful. Actually, we need not go back very far in time, since any physician trained in medicine before the discovery of penicillin would attest to how relatively unsophisticated medicine still was, even by the middle of the twentieth century. As one physician recalls,

> I graduated from medical school in 1938. Even in those days, medicine was more a priesthood than a science. A favorite examination question

> was, "If you are lost on a desert island with only six drugs, which drugs would suffice for good medical practice?" The answer was arsenicals for syphilis, quinine for malaria, insulin for diabetes, liver for pernicious anemia, digitalis for the heart, and morphine for pain. All other medicines were pure placebo. (Rosenbaum 1988: 198)

After the discovery of modern life-saving drugs, therapy dramatically improved in most aspects of medicine, to the extent that medicine has made more rapid and successful progress during the past 60 years than in the entire cumulative previous history of Western medicine, from Galen to the twentieth century.

Nevertheless, we do not yet have the answers to all medical questions, and in some significant areas we are hardly better informed about human behavior and medical practice than were ancient and medieval practitioners. Medicine remains an art, and tracing back the history of this art can help us better understand the processes of discovery and treatment.

Let us take one example, the problem of diet and health. Obesity has recently been recognized as one of the scourges of modern times, with little overall consensus as to how one should understand and act upon the issues involved. According to one expert, our modern ideas of diet were developed and promoted after the Second World War by the American Heart Association, based upon studies comparing cholesterol and heart attack rates in countries around the world. The research concluded that high levels of fat in modern diets were specifically responsible for obesity and heart disease, and recommended a low-fat, high-carbohydrate diet.[1] After a low-fat diet did not have the anticipated effect, new diets were introduced to improve health and reduce obesity, one requiring total fat restriction while another recommended exactly the opposite, a high-fat low-carbohydrate diet. Subsequent studies embraced contradictory advice, advocating diets based upon a theory of "good" and "bad" fats as well as "good" and "bad" carbohydrates (Agatston 2003: 16–21).

Our modern scientific world dispenses a great deal of confusing information about health and prevention of disease, which is a trait modern medicine shares with its ancient counterpart. Moreover, diets and trendy medications tend to be the obsessions of wealthier classes in society, and this situation hardly differs from antiquity, when the best medical advice was only on offer to those patients who could afford the costly services.

When we turn to ancient Babylonian medicine, one question often asked is whether any part of Babylonian medicine was actually effective. Did it work? We have hundreds of drugs cited in Babylonian medical recipes, in addition to long lists of plants and minerals used for medicinal purposes, often with descriptions of the drugs and of the diseases for which they could be used. We have no idea, however, how such data was compiled, since there were no clinical trials. How would ancient physicians know which plants were effective against which diseases? We can surmise that plants were identified over a very long period, perhaps going back to Neolithic times, and the use of such plants was determined by a hit-or-miss means of trying something to see what happens, and then keeping careful records of the results. The crucial point was to remember, later on, if the drug seemed to work.

One redeeming feature of Babylonian medicine is the lack of surgery, because of the substantial risks involved. Almost all Babylonian medical texts are limited to pharmacological preparations administered mostly as potions, salves, ointments, fumigations, or suppositories. Surgery would have been dangerous without either proper antiseptics or anesthesia, nor is there any firm evidence from Babylonia of bloodletting. For this reason, the Babylonian physician probably caused less harm to his patient than his later colleagues in medieval Europe.

Dissection and Disease Taxonomy

As we go back in time, the relationship between magic and medicine alters considerably, although not fundamentally. The technological basis for what we know as modern medicine has a long and tedious history, which actually made precious little advancement over many centuries. The major breakthrough leading to a scientific understanding of medicine came relatively late, in the fifteenth century, with dissection of the human body providing more precise knowledge of human anatomy. Meanwhile, autopsies were primarily an academic exercise, carried out exceptionally by some noted Greek physicians in Alexandria in the third century BC (von Staden 1998: 52). There are various practical reasons why the taboo of cutting open the human body was usually observed, even by Galen. First, before the invention of rubber gloves, dissection could have been dangerous since the researcher could easily contract a disease which had been the patient's cause of death (see Geller 2007: 187f.). Second, religious taboos no doubt played an important role, since disfiguring the human body was thought to have affected how the soul might appear in the afterlife. In Homer, for instance, the soldier in Hades is seen with his battle scars (Bernstein 1993: 30, 65). Apart from the taboo itself, the most probable reason for the lack of interest in dissection in ancient and medieval medicine was the fact that knowledge of internal anatomy did not actually help in healing the patient. Knowing where the organs were located and how the blood circulated were important discoveries in themselves, but how did one convert this knowledge into effective treatment?

It is not particularly easy to classify diseases within Babylonian medicine, although they fall generally within similar categories in Hippocratic medicine. Some diseases are simply associated with parts of the body, such as head disease, tooth disease, eye disease, nose disease, even foot disease, as well as kidney disease and anus disease. Baldness was treated as a disease. There are varieties of skin diseases, including rashes and pocks, as well as leprosy-like conditions affecting the nose and mouth, but it is impossible to diagnose these conditions according to modern disease terminology.

A major development in understanding disease only came with the discovery of morbid anatomy in the eighteenth century in Padua and at St George's Hospital, London, where physicians began to realize that autopsies after diagnosis could provide important clues to diagnosing disease correctly (Porter 1997: 263f.). It took centuries, however, for this idea to develop from the days of Egyptian mummification, which was the last period when dissections were carried out on a regular basis as part of embalming, or from third-century BC Alexandria, where a few Greek physicians practiced vivisection on prisoners.

What this effectively means is that ancient and medieval medicine had much in common, and that the fundamental relationship between doctor and patient remained fairly constant over the centuries. The relationship between magic and medicine – the psychological and technical approaches to healing – was always present and was constantly evolving. We will see that although real technological advancement in medicine was slow in developing, knowledge about disease and healing improved over time, and theories about disease and healing were changing as well. Not every new idea is an advancement or an improvement on what came before, but the complex relationship between magic and medicine is usually affected by new theories of healing, or even by skepticism towards accepted theories.

Another factor determining how magic and medicine relate to each other is the complex relationship between doctor and patient, in the ancient world as in our own society. Within Mesopotamia, there is much we do not know about this relationship. Was the doctor paid, and how much? What was his status within society? Would men and women be

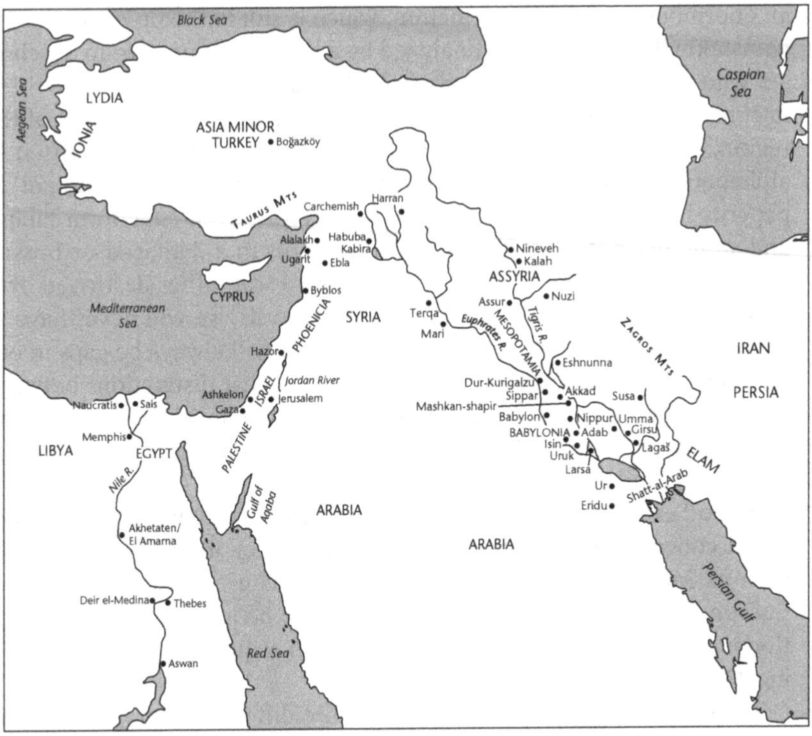

Map 1 The Near East (Mark W. Chavalas, *The Ancient Near East*, Blackwell, 2006)

treated by the same doctor? Was medical help readily available? How many doctors were there within a community, or was medicine only available to the royal household and those closely associated with either the palace or temple? Although there is much here that we would like to know but will probably never know, it is possible to make some reasonable assumptions based upon the data which we have. But first, it is important to clarify the nature of our sources.

The Sources

Mesopotamian society is better documented over the three millennia than any other ancient society, including Egypt. The many thousands of cuneiform tablets which survive because of the durability of clay provide an enormous wealth of information, which is still in the process of being painstakingly collected and analyzed by a relatively small group of scholars who read Sumerian, Akkadian, Hittite, and other languages written in cuneiform script. We also have much data from other languages of the region, such as Aramaic, Phoenician, Ugaritic, and Hebrew, written in alphabetic scripts, although anything written on either parchment or papyrus had a much poorer chance of survival. Even cuneiform tablets and stone inscriptions often come down to us in a damaged or broken state, and much of the ancient written record was either destroyed over time or remains to be discovered. In other words, we will never have as much information as we would like and there will always be gaps in our knowledge. This means that we have to make clear distinctions between evidence and inference, by noting what information we have in the form of written or pictographic records, and then being direct about what inferences can be drawn from this data.

A good example of evidence versus inference as applied to the ancient world concerns the debate over levels of literacy in an ancient society such as Mesopotamia. The model we tend to use is that of medieval Europe, where levels of literacy are known to be low. The usual assumption is that scribes performed all tasks which required reading and writing. Does the same apply to Mesopotamia?

The evidence from Mesopotamia is quite different from what we find in medieval Europe (see Charpin 2004: 31ff.; Cryer 1994: 138–41). The many thousands of cuneiform tablets dealing with simple transactions, such as loans or purchases, deeds, contracts, letters, and receipts, indicate that there was a sophisticated urban economy, usually based upon the activities of the palace or temple, as well as the business interests of important commercial families. The many documents show a great variety of handwriting, from very formal to very cursive, and from sophisticated accountancy records to simple receipts. One could infer from this data that professional scribes were responsible for all these written records, and that the general population remained illiterate.[2] Moreover, since two prominent kings, Assurbanipal and Nabonidus, boasted of their skills in the art of writing, one jumps to the conclusion that *only* these two kings in first-millennium Assyria and Babylonia were literate (Beaulieu 2007: 473). Several factors argue against this point of view.

In the first instance, we usually assume that cuneiform script was difficult to learn,[3] much more difficult, in fact, than learning an alphabet. The assumption is that the 600-odd cuneiform-sign repertoire of Sumerian and Akkadian was too cumbersome for traders and merchants, who ultimately invented a much simpler writing system – the alphabet – which then spread throughout the world. By simply inventing a system of writing consonants rather than vowels, the "original" alphabet boiled down a 600-odd character system into 30 characters or fewer, and this new system of writing is thought to have facilitated the spread of literacy.

If we separate evidence and inference, things appear somewhat differently. It is true that the alphabet drastically reduced the number of characters for writing languages. Nevertheless, the assumption that an alphabet is easier to read than a cuneiform syllabary needs to be challenged.[4] It is not easier. For a native speaker of Akkadian, learning to write cuneiform only required a knowledge of some 100 basic signs, and these signs are clearly phonetic (see also Charpin 2004: 52–60). This means that one has a different sign for BA, BU, BI, or MA, MU, MI, as well as AB or AM, or even BAB. The phonetic nature of the script, once one learns the signs, makes it quite easy to write Akkadian or even to read the Akkadian of a simple business document or private letter. Of course one had to be much better educated in the scribal schools to read more sophisticated court letters, literature, astronomical texts, medical texts, etc., but this is just as true today as then. Second, it is not necessarily easier to read an alphabet as such, despite the fact that it has many fewer characters, since the reader must supply the vowels in order to sound out the script accurately, and readings are not always obvious. The script is not phonetic. Furthermore, the invention of the alphabet did not immediately occasion the abandonment of cuneiform scripts, which kept being used for almost two millennia after the introduction of the alphabet.

There is one other factor which may reflect the levels of literacy in Mesopotamia, namely the easy availability of writing materials. Cuneiform tablets were essentially cost-free, with clay easily available, and the stylus made of reed. Papyrus was relatively cheap but still had to be rolled and treated to make a sheet of writing materials, and writing required ink. Parchment was expensive, being made from animal hide. It is quite plausible, therefore, that once a Babylonian could master the mechanics of reading and writing simple cuneiform without too much difficulty, writing materials were easy to come by, and these two factors encouraged the spread of literacy.

The emergence of writing in Mesopotamia may have also been influenced by the context of an urban rather a predominantly rural society. Large cities, such as Eridu and Uruk, can be traced back to prehistoric Mesopotamia of the fourth millennium BC. Other large cities developed along the alluvial plain of the Tigris and Euphrates, and these cities depended upon a highly developed system of dikes and canals for controlling irrigation, which was made possible through the use of a large corvée of workers controlled by a central bureaucracy. The landscape itself encouraged the development of urban culture, and the rivers were used as major highways for transporting goods (Algaze 2008: 51ff.). Already by the third millennium BC, we see a society characterized by widespread trading contacts, large-scale building complexes, great walled cities, and many different types of professional and artisan classes. The literature of the time also shows a preference for urban life, viewing the open countryside between cities as hostile territory rife with bandits and demons.

In effect, magical and medical literature from Mesopotamia originates from a relatively literate and urban society, in which some form of medical expertise, offered by either an exorcist, physician, midwife, or barber, was probably available to anyone, either at the temple or in a shop or stall on the street. This may explain the differences in our magic and medical tablets, which range from clear library handwritings, often in many columns, to small tablets in cursive scripts preserving a single prescription or a simple magical spell. There were probably many different healers for different clients, depending upon their social status, wealth, or gender, and perhaps even specialists for different types of medical problems.

Is Medicine Magic and Is Magic Medicine?

In Babylonia, both magic and medicine served as strategies for healing the sick, marshaling the authority of religion whenever possible. The great English scholar Reginald Campbell Thompson published copies and editions and translations of Babylonian medical texts throughout the 1920s and 1930s, but he never attempted a synthesis explaining how the system actually worked and what made Babylonian medicine tick. The French scholar Rene Labat gave us an edition of the Babylonian manual of diagnosis and prognosis, but his publication made surprisingly little impact on the world of history of medicine, despite presenting much relevant material (Labat 1951). What was obvious from these early studies was that Babylonian medicine contained a fair amount of magic: incantations appeared alongside recipes within the medical corpus, and diseases were often thought to have been brought on by various gods and demons. The vast majority of Babylonian medical texts were published in cuneiform copy only by Franz Köcher from Berlin, which included many texts which could be classified as magico-medicine, inhabiting the grey area between pure magic and pure medicine.

In fact, the complex relationship between magic and medicine persisted within all systems of healing in the ancient and medieval world, although this relationship differs over the course of centuries as healing methods changed and improved. The psychological dimensions of therapy or healing arts, which we will refer to as "magic," have always played an important role within the practice of treatments which we know of as "medicine." This fluid relationship between magic and medicine is dynamic, depending upon the level of sophistication of healing therapies. Our attitudes towards magic and medicine today are quite different than those of our great-grandparents, who lived before the invention of penicillin and the invention of drugs which can prolong life. Even today, the patient often feels better once he enters the doctor's surgery, and the sight of the doctor's white coat and stethoscope makes an impression on the patient which become part of the healing process.

Our use of the terms "magic" and "medicine" is somewhat misleading, since ancient Babylonian scholars used no such terminology. Healing therapy consisted of a combination of therapeutic recipes and incantations, since recipes were often accompanied by incantations. One modern approach to Babylonian magic and medicine avoids any categorical distinctions between incantations and medical recipes as separate genres, but treats each type of text as a form of "therapy," usually for different types of illnesses. Incantations are essentially appeals to the psychology of the patient, while medical recipes treat symptoms such as fever, pain, diarrhea, and other physical signs of disease, using potions, pills, salves, ointments, pessaries and suppositories, etc. At the same time, there is also ample evidence that exorcists could treat physical illnesses (Schramm 2008: 26f.; Böck 2007: 175; Jean 2006: 166), while "medicine" could use *materia medica* against mental illness.[5]

The overlap between these two complementary methods of healing – recipes and incantations – are different means of achieving similar ends. Incantations frequently appearing in medical recipes provided the patient with confidence that the therapy itself had divine sanction and precedence and would work. Healing rituals used with incantations, in non-recipe contexts, provided for fumigations and massage as alternative means for purifying and healing substances to be applied to the patient. According to this approach, there is no need to assign one set of therapies to an artificial category – magic – and the other to another equally artificial category – medicine.

We can also attempt to imagine the situation from the patient's perspective: how did one choose between visiting the exorcist and visiting the physician? On what did this decision depend, and was it a free choice or was it determined by social or economic considerations (for which we have little evidence)? Perhaps, by the late first millennium, it made little difference, because an exorcist would have known enough about medicine (in its basic forms) or the physician would have known enough about incantations to be able to handle most ailments. On the other hand, there may have been a difference between primary care and specialist care, which we cannot judge from the evidence; did a patient first visit an exorcist or a doctor? One final possibility is that a patient (who could afford to do so) would ideally visit *both* exorcist and physician, for treatments covering the full range of physical and psychological conditions. Later systems of medicine paid due attention to both mind and body; Maimonides, for instance, later advocated a balanced state of mind as well as a strict regimen for optimal health.

The scope of the present study examines how medicine (and to a lesser extent, magic) evolved in Babylonia at the end of a long period of gestation and development, during a period extending over some 2000 years. It is not possible to trace every aspect of this development, since many things change over two millennia, including social and political milieux as well as basic scientific knowledge, apart from possible influences from elsewhere (Egypt and Greece). Our task will be to examine the end product of this process, to view state of the art Babylonian medicine in its final period of maturity, in the second half of the first millennium BC.

1

Medicine as Science

Scientific theory and epistemology are normally reckoned as the great discovery of the Greeks. Thales, Euclid, Hippocrates, Aristotle, and many other thinkers from Greece and Asia Minor are considered to have launched a great intellectual revolution, which created a specific kind of "scientific" thinking. This revolution is thought to be the basis for modern science, and especially natural sciences. The intellectual potential of Babylonian thinkers, on the other hand, with their own type of wisdom, is evaluated in very different terms: Babylonians are usually thought to have hardly indulged in theory but limited themselves to pragmatic and practical speculation about the physical world, without reference to hypothetical generalizations or methodological rules. Within the realm of medicine, for instance, Babylonians are known to have had no "theory of humors," as had the Greeks, and Babylonians saw diseases as being caused by demons and magical agents. This naturally has led to the conclusion that Babylonian medicine was unscientific, or at least less scientific than that of the Greeks.

It is true that Babylonian thinkers have left us no theoretical works among the many thousands of surviving cuneiform tablets from Mesopotamia; philosophy was simply not a Babylonian literary genre. This does not mean, however, that philosophical arguments were unknown to Babylonian scribal schools or scholars, but that philosophical writing was not part of the cuneiform repertoire. On the other hand, it is hardly conceivable that a complicated system of medicine like that used in Babylonia could have functioned devoid of theory. The problem is how to recognize and disinter Babylonian epistemology and theory from within the array of sources at our disposal.

The view taken here is that "theory" within an ancient context requires three necessary preconditions, in order to identify what we would consider to be rational but non-technological thinking. These three preconditions are: *imagination*, *deductive logic*, and *observation*. Let us take each in turn.

Imagination: Ancient science sought to find a general explanation for natural occurrences, with one general aim, namely to reduce the impression of randomness of what happens around us. There were countless numbers of events which imparted a feeling of "randomness" (in the way that quantum physics uses this term) among ancient peoples, such as movements of stars, changes in weather and climate, infinite variations and changes among flora and fauna, etc. The structure of this universal explanation is ambitious, namely the search for the simple (and generally valid) clarification of an endless number of happenings being brought about by a limited number of causes. In this way, the overwhelming randomness of the universe can be reduced to a relatively few factors.

Deductive logic: Babylonian epistemology bases itself upon logical deduction in which general patterns can be inferred from a myriad of details. A typical example of this kind of deduction can be seen in the relationship between the protasis and apodosis clauses of omens. The basic formulation of all Babylonian omens is, "if so-and-so happens, then so-and-so *can* result" (see Rochberg 2004: 257–9). Omens offer a strategy for counteracting a notion of randomness by reducing a great many "signs" into a relatively small number of results; even if gods ultimately control what happens, the patterns of signs or omens limit the number of possible explanations for otherwise seemingly random events.

As soon as one can find probable connections between, for example, a celestial event and corresponding incidents on earth, one can establish a system of quasi-causality for many different phenomena, thereby explaining otherwise seemingly arbitrary and haphazard occurrences. This is why Babylonian scholars developed a "database" of omens and signs in a system designed to infer and predict what would happen in the future based upon previous experience. If omen A was associated with event B at some time in the past, inference would suggest that the reoccurrence of A *might* lead to the reoccurrence of B. From a modern perspective, the entire logic is fallacious, and we would dismiss the association of two seemingly unrelated events as the fallacy of "post hoc ergo propter hoc," namely the fallacy of assuming that where two events are in sequence the second is caused by the first.[6] Nevertheless, we must admit that this type of deductive logic in Babylonia was not entirely without purpose, since establishing a relationship between data and inference is after all the beginning of methodical and scientific thinking.

Observation: In order for "observation" to qualify as a tool of science, the process must be formalized and calibrated. Rather than casual viewing, scientific observation must be periodic and regular with results being recorded. Babylonian scholars systematically collected an enormous quantity of data and information about the world around them, organized into relatively simple classifications, listing ordinary household objects, plants, stones, stars, as well as gods and illnesses; other lists recorded all kinds of ominous events in the world, based upon movements of celestial bodies and birds, climate and weather patterns, the shape and appearance of internal organs of animals, and much more. Classification and taxonomy are crucial ways of bringing order into a seemingly chaotic universe (see Veldhuis 1997: 2–8).

A large part of scientific thinking concerns observations of actions and reactions in the natural world, although ancient man had virtually no instrumentation or technology available to him (apart from simple measuring tools) in order to try to establish causality between two reacting phenomena. One of the main characteristics of ancient scientific thinking is the general failure of ancient savants to validate the results or conclusions of others. Claims were never systematically checked, but everything was based upon the authority of the claimant. This was as true of the Greco-Roman world as in the Orient; a common rhetorical device used by the Romans in courts of law was to discount the observations of others by questioning the authority of the person making the observation, rather than by checking the facts,[7] a technique also employed by Galen.

"Scientific" Medicine

The three characteristics – *imagination, deductive logic,* and *observation* – are postulated as the essential intellectual basis for all ancient science, whether in Babylon or Athens. These same three prerequisites to scientific thinking are also to be found within the framework of Babylonian medicine, although in somewhat different forms.[8] We would redefine these three intellectual characteristics within Babylonian medicine in the following categories.

First, the function of *imagination* corresponds within Babylonian medicine to a related factor: magic. One might qualify this statement somewhat: the function of imagination corresponds to any phenomenon within Babylonian medicine which we would call "magic." We have already referred to the problem of "randomness," which needed to be addressed by Babylonian as well as every other system of ancient medicine. Magic offered a solution. There were and still are obvious questions relating to randomness, such as "Why am I sick and not my neighbor?" "Why do I have pain in my head/stomach/foot, and nowhere else?" "Why this illness and not some other?" "What has caused this illness?" The countless number of possibilities can be dramatically reduced by what we call "magic."

The system worked as follows: in the Babylonian view of the world, gods decided all matters dealing with human fate. Babylonian scholars grounded much of their scientific knowledge in an ancient belief system incorporating magic, in which illnesses were ultimately caused by demons or angry gods, or perhaps indirectly caused by these same factors through, for example, ingesting bewitched foodstuffs. This belief system formed a useful general background explanation for the ultimate causes of illness, which the patient could readily accept. This general explanation of illness, however, would never be expounded as theory per se in any Babylonian tractate. On the other hand, in comparison with the Greek theory of "humors," the Babylonian idea of demons as invisible bearers of disease conforms in some ways more closely to modern notions of bacteria and viruses. Babylonian medicine in this respect may not be less rational than a Greek conception that disease was caused by internal bodily imbalances.

In fact, Greek schools of medicine held contradictory views concerning the causes of illness.[9] Hippocrates was not the only doctor in town. In contrast to the Hippocratics, the ancient Greek world knew other philosophies of medicine, such as Methodists and Empiricists, who argued that the search for causes of disease was a distraction preventing the physician from investigating a proper cure. According to this opposing view, an effective cure was much more valuable than philosophical speculation about the potential causes of disease. In certain respects, the Methodists correctly evaluated the limitations of ancient medicine by insisting on a more practical approach to healing, pointing out that a philosophical theory of disease had only limited application to the actual healing of patients. Surprisingly, the Methodists, in the second century BC, introduced into the Greco-Roman world a type of medical practice which more-or-less resembled that of contemporary Babylonia, which concentrated on practice and recipes to the exclusion of theory. The growth of these anti-Hippocratic medical philosophies may have coincided with an increased general skepticism in the Roman world, as exemplified by the rise of the Skeptic school of philosophy, as well as fitting in with a general objection to all things Greek, as forcefully expounded by Cato the Elder (Nutton 2004: 148, 162). As Owsei Temkin observes, "the methodist sect, because of its practical orientation and disdain of complicated theories, appealed to the temper of the Roman people" (Temkin 1956: xxix).

The role of *deductive logic* and analogy in Babylonian medical thinking (our second category) needs further clarification. Beyond a general notion of ultimate causation of disease as a result of divine disfavor or simply fate, Babylonian medicine developed its own system for relating diseases to symptoms in a quasi-causal relationship. The logic was essentially the same as that for numerous types of Babylonian omens, as discussed above, and a formal system of recording omens and potents was adopted by Babylonian medicine for diagnosis and prognosis (Oppenheim 1977: 224). In effect, symptoms became omens. The omen apodoses were prognostic, used to determine whether the patient would continue to live or die, and if the latter, when? After three days? Four days? Within a month?

There is a difference, however, between medical prognostic omens and all other types of omens. The difference is that the connection between the protasis and apodosis of medical prognostic omens is based upon a reality not to be found in other types of omen literature (Oppenheim 1977: 294). In other words, in the case of medical omens, results were potentially capable of being substantiated or refuted. Ancient physicians, for instance, were capable of estimating for how long a certain fever was likely to last, or how life-threatening or dangerous a certain infection was likely to be, simply by repeated experience of observing fevers of the same type. The "post hoc ergo propter hoc" fallacy of other types of omens cannot be applied in the same way to the medical omens, since the connection between data and inferences was likely to be more realistic, and one could note what actually *happened* after the occurrence of a sign, symptom, or "omen." In other words, medical omens could reflect real observations of "action-reaction" situations, the connection between disease as a cause (of changes in the body) and symptom as a sign (of changes in the body), while other types of omens could not make the same claim to causality.[10]

This brings us to our third point, namely *observation* as a function of epistemology. Since actual instruments (e.g. thermometers and stethoscopes) were unavailable then, ancient physicians were entirely dependent upon observation.[11] Within the framework of medicine, we must include an additional factor, namely "experience," best understood in the

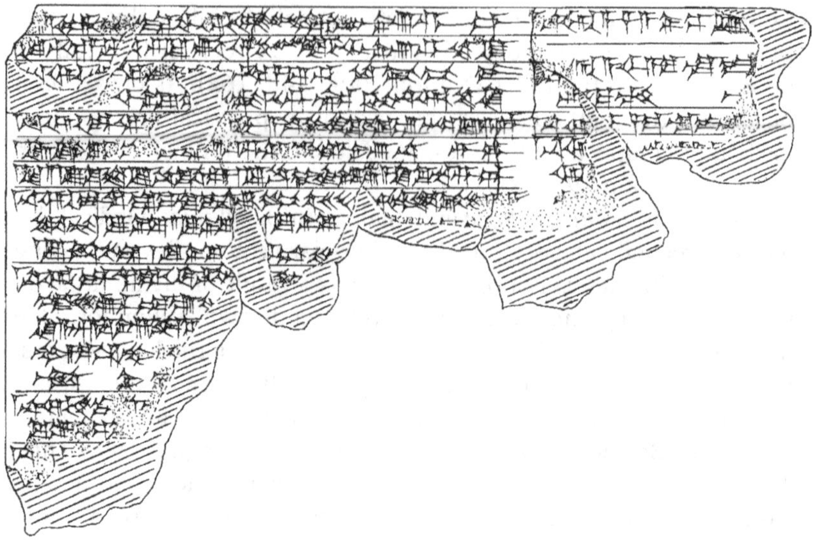

Figure 1.1 Medical tablet from Babylon mentioning Hammurapi's mother (BM 41293+44866; copy M. J. Geller)

French equivalent term *expérience* also denoting "experiment." As Roger French comments regarding Alexandrian medicine, "experience was now not only a question of personal observation, but the experience of others, which could be read in books."[12] We need to explore how this combination of "observation" and "experience" actually functioned.

A medical tablet from Babylon, dated roughly to the latter half of the first millennium BC, has an unusual opening line in what is otherwise quite an ordinary medical recipe for eye disease (see Figure 1.1). The tablet begins with the line, "[If] Hammurapi's mother suffered from eye disease …".[13] The *Vorlage* of this tablet was obviously broken at this point, as noted by the scribe himself, and the actual symptoms ascribed to Hammurabi's mother were not preserved at the time the tablet was copied.[14] The rest of the tablet contains eye-disease recipes which are known from other Late Assyrian and Late Babylonian sources (see Fincke 2000: 86–91). The scribe himself was no doubt copying from an older manuscript containing eye-disease recipes, but whether the original manuscript was actually from the time of Hammurabi himself is doubtful. Why should this tablet refer to Hammurabi's mother, who lived some 1500 years before this tablet was being copied? The most likely explanation is that the scribe was referring back to a celebrated case of eye disease which was recorded and remembered in a much later era. A similar case of retrospective attribution of medical recipes to a venerable old tradition occurs in an unusual colophon of a tablet devoted to fever occurring in the brain. The colophon reads:

> Proven and tested salves and poultices, fit for use, from the mouth of ancient antediluvian sages from Šuruppak, which Enlil-muballiṭ, sage (*apkallu*) of Nippur, left (to posterity) in the second year of Enlil-bani, king of Isin.[15] (*AMT* 105; see Hunger 1968: No. 533)

Although the tablet itself is not earlier than the eighth century BC, the poultice is attributed to oral transmitted medical lore dating back to c. 1860 BC, more than a millennium earlier, and ultimately to mythological sages from before the Flood;[16] nothing could be more authoritative. This particular colophon goes further in stating that experience gathered over a very long period of time, from ancient experts to contemporary physicians, makes these poultices tried and true. In the absence of clinical trials, generations of usage of drugs effectively acted as a filter to determine which drugs were effective (and which not).[17]

There is nothing particularly unusual about a medical tablet colophon claiming that a recipe is "tried and tested," although we are not given any indication of the testing process.[18] Occasionally tablets attest to the effectiveness of the drugs mentioned, such as an Assur tablet serving as the equivalent of a modern Physician's Desk Reference listing various measures of common drugs, with the following appended note:

> This lotion is effective and tested against jaundice and hepatitis. Lotion of oils (for) "sun-fever." (*BAM* 186: 10–13 [cuneiform text only])

We have no way of knowing what exactly is meant by "effective and tested," except the authority of the well-known Assur *mašmaššu*, Kiṣir-Assur, who "hastily excerpted" the recipe and wrote the tablet. What we have here is a good example of "experience," in which the scholar or physician brings to mind an earlier successful formula or treatment, which was noted and recorded. Vivian Nutton has found a similar approach within Greek medicine:

> Case histories, the codified record of previous success, played an important role, providing a wider data bank for future use. The Empiricists were particularly keen on recording information on drugs and their effectiveness. … The weakness of experience … was that it dealt only with the past: when faced with an apparently new condition or new circumstances … the Empiricist doctor had to start effectively from scratch and resort to a

> method of trial and error. Such criticism was countered by the principle that, having observed carefully the conditions of any case, the doctor should choose whatever therapy had worked in "similar" circumstances. (Nutton 2004: 148)

Academic Medicine

Babylonian science in the latter half of the first millennium BC formed an integral part of the school curriculum (Gesche 2001: 213–16; Hunger 1976) and these disciplines were characterized by large collections of data which were then studied and analyzed, in an attempt to explain many aspects of the physical world. Although mathematics, astronomy and astrology, medicine, magic, and divination do not all conform to our modern notions of "science," they nevertheless need to be perceived in terms of their methodologies and how they assembled data, as well as their applications to everyday life.

We wonder whether Babylonians, in the course of collecting data on physical and perceived phenomena of their world, could have invented a rudimentary "scientific method" which might be comparable to scientific thinking today (Rochberg 2004: 96f.); the same question has been directed towards Greek science (Russo 2004: 21ff.). Babylonians for most of their history inhabited a world which was mostly devoid of technology, and the symbiosis of mechanics and science came later. Babylonians had few instruments for measurements or calculation, and virtually no telescopes or microscopes, or navigational instruments.

Of course technology is not a *sine qua non* for scientific thinking, since mental models can be used as tools for investigating physics, as has been demonstrated for Greek science (Renn and Damerow 2007), and for Babylonian mathematics (Damerow 2007). In the same way, we can investigate Babylonian "sciences" (including medicine, magic, and divination) as intellectual disciplines, with one caveat. We will impose a rule of thumb, that the more "mathematical" a Babylonian discipline tends to be, the more "scientific" in our modern sense. Let us give a few examples below.

Mathematics, on *a priori* grounds, yields the best results as a scientific form of thinking. Although it has usually been understood that Babylonians developed little in the way of mathematical theorems or hypotheses, recent studies have shown that Babylonian scholars certainly understood and taught mathematics in a way which showed that they grasped the rudiments of Euclidian mathematics long before Euclid (Friberg 2007; but see Robson 2008: 281f.).

The next important burst of scientific discovery occurred before the middle of the first millennium BC, when astronomers in Babylon began to make much more accurate charts of the movements of stars and planets in relation to each other and to the sun and moon, to the extent that accurate predictions became possible. In this regard, complex calculations of heavenly phenomena became increasingly important and moved mathematics on from its close association with algebraic geometry, with its origin in surveying of fields. The need to have mathematics serve the needs of astronomy may have given it a vital boost and even generated a new interest in mathematics, after the heyday of mathematics in the Old Babylonian period of the second millennium BC. This dramatic change in the need for new types of calculations can easily go unnoticed, since we have no mathematical or school texts which are designed to illustrate the logic of mathematical astronomy. Furthermore, the study of mathematics appears to have gone into decline by the mid-second millennium BC, lying dormant for nearly a millennium.

By the mid-first millennium BC mathematical astronomy had become fundamental. Its calculations were basic tools of astronomy and served to kick-start mathematics within the school curriculum once again. Significant Babylonian advances in astronomy began taking place, based on an essential mathematical component, to provide accurate predictions of the movements of the moon, constellations, and planets, as well as eclipses. The zodiac first appears in Achaemenid Babylonia and was adopted by Greek astrology. Aside from mathematics, astronomical data was gathered by daily observation of the heavens, recorded in "astronomical diaries" providing information about the moon, sun, and planets, solstices and equinoxes, meteors and comets, the weather, market prices of certain commodities, the height of the Euphrates, and occasionally a significant historic event on the day, usually involving the king. The calculations of time intervals used in the diaries were probably based on the use of a water-clock, and the diaries are remarkable for the accuracy of the recorded data.

Materia Medica

The combination of observation and experience certainly benefited Babylonian therapy, which governed the use of plants and drugs in medical recipes. The epistemological question is how Babylonian scholars managed to recognize the chemical effects of plants, without the benefit of laboratories or clinical trials. Nevertheless, they studied, listed, and categorized plants and minerals under a specific classification system, which they labeled with the Akkadian word *šiknu*, meaning "nature" or "character," e.g. "the *šiknu* of a plant/stone is …".[19] This term *šiknu* is significant since the Greeks used the term *physis*, "nature," in a similar sense, although such terminology is by no means universal in other systems of ancient medicine.[20]

The question therefore remains, how Babylonians could have discovered the effective properties of plants and minerals and what effect they would have upon the human body. That the Babylonians did indeed have some idea of what changes plants and minerals were capable of producing in the body can be seen from Akkadian therapeutic texts themselves, which distinguish between "simple" and "complex" recipes. A "simple" is a recipe which employs a single-ingredient drug against a single illness.[21] We also find, on the other hand, numerous cases of complex recipes composed of combinations of plants, minerals, and other ingredients, used as panaceas against one or more diseases.

We are far from understanding Babylonian medical recipes because we can only identify with accuracy relatively few of the ingredients. The dosage and amounts of the drugs also remain unclear to us. Hence, for the moment, drafting a proper taxonomy of Babylonian drugs is a hopeless enterprise, nor can adequate comparisons be made with the works of Dioscorides and Theophrastus, in which plant and mineral names are much better understood than those of their Babylonian counterparts.[22] Nevertheless, some general features of Babylonian recipes can be noted. Babylonian physicians made clear typological distinctions between recipes aimed at specific ailments. For example, rectal-disease texts employed much more oil in recipes, while kidney-disease texts employed more minerals, and eye-disease recipes used more salves. Babylonian physicians had worked out a system for the use of simple and complex drugs, which we do not yet fully comprehend.[23]

The great bulk of Babylonian medical recipes are concerned with pharmacological methods of alleviating symptoms, and there is quite a variety of methods for drugs to be administered. One of the most effective methods of administering drugs was through fumigation, by which drugs were inhaled and could rapidly be absorbed into the bloodstream.

The *materia medica* of Babylonian recipes consisted of trees and plant matter (seeds, roots, sprouts, leaves, fruit, branches, even wood), grains such as barley and flour, and various spices and vegetables. There was a variety of liquids into which drugs could be dissolved, such as water, milk, fish brine, sesame oil, and urine, and in some cases drugs were filtered and distilled; alcohol (beer and wine) were excellent agents for dissolving drugs. In many cases, drugs could be mixed with animal products such as sheep fat and lard, and less regularly in fish brine, blood, and bone marrow. Some exotic animal products were also used as *materia medica*, such as mongoose blood, turtle and mussel shells, and other animal viscera. Mineral stones could also be ground up, and the recipes call for animal or even human excrement (e.g. bat guano), but such *Dreckapotheke* have been shown to be secret names for ordinary plants (Köcher 1995).

Once the plants or other items have been gathered, there is a long list of how they must be treated and used to make up the recipes themselves: *materia medica* need to be "taken" in the first instance (i.e. gathered or selected), then weighed, washed, immersed, dried and desiccated, roasted and burned, crushed, pounded, cut up, beaten, diced, chopped, grated, pulverized, sifted, pressed out, soaked and dissolved, kneaded, stirred, sprinkled, saturated, spread, blended and mixed, poured out into vessels, warmed up and heated in an oven, cooked and boiled, and finally cooled. Each of these actions is governed by a rich and varied medical technical vocabulary (see Goltz 1974: index), with parallels in Greek medical recipes. Drugs, consisting mostly of plants and minerals, were prepared in the form of potions, salves, powders, pills, tampons, and pessaries, to be ingested, rubbed onto the body, applied as a bandage, or inserted into the anus, urethra, ears, or vagina through lubricated copper tubes or reeds. Not only was there a large variety of drugs, but there was an equally important variety of ways in which drugs could be utilized, in both simples and compound recipes.

Anatomical Science

Anatomy posed serious problems, even for experienced doctors, since neither Babylonians nor Hippocratics engaged in dissection or autopsy on human corpses. Babylonians, like Greeks, had little actual knowledge of workings of the internal anatomy, except for that gleaned from comparisons with animal physiognomy. Only in the third century BC did Greek scholars in Alexandria, Herophilus and Erasistratos,[24] indulge in human vivisection, but this revolutionary approach to medicine was short-lived.[25]

Egypt, of course, had a clear potential advantage in the field of anatomical knowledge, due to the practice of mummification, in which the main internal organs were extracted and placed into canopic jars. This does not mean, however, that such knowledge was widespread or even generally appreciated. Judging from the extant Egyptian medical corpus, it is far from clear whether funerary experts mummifying bodies transmitted the fruits of their anatomical experience to Egyptian doctors (Nunn 1996: 43f., 65), and in any case embalming had little to do with medicine in Egypt (von Staden 1998: 29). In general, prior to the third century BC no scholars in antiquity had any real understanding of internal human anatomy.

In Babylonia, much more was known about the internal anatomy of sheep than humans, judging by the very precise terminology for internal sheep organs that can be found in divination texts. Although we have no single Akkadian word specifically designating the human heart,[26] Babylonian diviners identified no less than eight different areas of a sheep's heart (see Geller 2007: 188f.). Moreover, there is no clear evidence that diviners and physicians ever compared notes during the formative periods when Babylonian medicine was taking shape, in the Old Babylonian period in the first half of the second millennium BC. By the Hellenistic period, exorcists became the scholars responsible for copying and recording divination texts (Robson 2008: 241f.), but this knowledge does not seem to have spurred on any new Babylonian studies of human anatomy. Nevertheless, despite the fact that the physician's observations were limited to the external anatomy of his patients, the combination of observation and experience led to some impressive results. Physicians were able to observe cases of "action-reaction," namely what specific changes came about in the body which were caused by disease.[27]

Medical Predictions

By the mid-first millennium BC, the increased ability of Babylonian astronomers to make accurate predictions had a putative influence upon other sciences as well. The problem with other disciplines, such as medicine or magic, was the lack of any real mathematical basis for predictions regarding the physical and mental health of patients. Medics and magicians tried to introduce astral medicine and astral magic into their own calculations, hoping that the accuracy of predicting the appearance of planets might transfer over into predicting the onslaught or course of disease. Although previously celestial divination and omens had traditionally focused on the changing positions of constellations and planets, or the sun and moon, to make general predictions about plagues or epidemics, the new astral medicine relied upon the zodiac and more accurate predictions of celestial motion to try to determine which specific diseases and treatments in individual patients were likely to be affected by celestial phenomena.

To determine the "scientific quotient" of Babylonian medicine, based upon our rule of thumb about a mathematical component, we should look at aspects of Babylonian medicine which demonstrate rudimentary scientific thinking, unaided by instruments. Babylonian healers were adept at observing symptoms of patients and recording them scrupulously. One of the staples of Babylonian therapy, the lengthy list of symptoms comprising the so-called Diagnostic Handbook (Labat 1951; Heeßel 2000), allows us but few insights into ancient disease taxonomy, since symptoms were not assigned to the diseases which generated them, but rather to the parts of the human body which exhibited these symptoms. There is virtually no evidence that symptom lists were compiled from case histories, but they were largely a conglomeration of symptoms drawn from many different patients, for the purpose of describing disease in general and not illnesses associated with any single individual. Nevertheless, in terms of scientific thinking the Diagnostic Handbook represents one method for collecting and analyzing data, even if the underlying assumptions of the process do not conform to modern notions of diagnosis.[28]

Three examples of diagnostic texts will help to illustrate these texts, with the first being an example of symptoms taken from the temples of the head:

> If (a man's) temples are under pressure and he is hot (and) cold: hand of Kūbu.
> If the temples are under pressure and his internal organs move: hand of Kūbu.
> If the temples are under pressure and his internal organs keep swelling up: hand of Kūbu.
> If the temples are under pressure and his ears do not hear (anything): hand of his personal god being laid on him, he will die.
> If his temple is in good shape, he will recover; if his temple collapses, he will die. (Labat 1951: 32–3, 1–5)

The symptoms are described in a methodical but mechanical way, with no indication of the individual characteristics of a patient, or an awareness of other symptoms that might occur. The crucial question being addressed here is whether the patient will live or die, a concern that is also found in Diagnostic Handbook symptoms derived from the patient's face:

> If (a man's) face is covered with a yellow paste, his lips are covered with a film, his eyes secrete yellow (stuff), and his right eye squints, he will die.
> If his face is deformed, he will die.
> If his face is deformed and his tongue is yellow, (in fact) his body is yellow, he is ill in the stomach and will die (latest) on the third day. (Labat 1951: 74–5, 29–31)

Similar prognostic texts are known from aphorisms in the Hippocratic corpus (e.g. Lloyd 1983: 171). Not all passages demonstrate this pattern:

> If a man's complexion changes, his eyes roll around, his eyes begin to squint, he constantly scratches his lips and his chin, blood flows from his nose without being able to staunch it: the Gallû-demon has seized this man. (After Labat 1951: 190–91, 14; see *Iraq* 19: 40)

This passage (from the end of the composition) describes a group of different head symptoms and also provides a diagnosis; the attack of the Gallû-demon designates a certain type of illness. As with all other examples of the Diagnostic Handbook, we have no way of knowing in how many patients these same symptoms were noted, but such a passage is unlikely to be based on a single case history.

Medical Prescriptions

The largest genre of medical texts from Babylon were therapeutic texts, which begin with a symptom and then list drugs and procedures designed to relieve the symptoms (but not necessarily cure the disease). It is likely that a cure for disease was considered to be the province of gods (to be approached though magic and incantations, through an exorcist), while the physician's role was to treat symptoms. Among texts with a high "scientific quotient," therapeutic texts get a higher score than magical incantations, partly because of the mathematics rule of thumb we have been using (i.e. the more math, the more "science"). Therapeutic texts erratically (and not always) provide amounts or weights of each ingredient in a recipe, presumably reflecting relative proportions of ingredients, and occasionally give information about dosage, e.g. drugs to be administered three times a day, etc. Consider the following:

> If ditto (= diseased anus), grind up 5 *sila* of flax seed, sieve, and you steep it in milk,
> bind (it) for 14 days on the chest and shoulder and he will improve; the ingredients [are checked].
>
> ---
>
> When you have tied on these poultices on him, he drinks 1/3 *sila* of date-juice, 10 *kisal*-weight of oil and afterwards he should not drink any [other] drug; he keeps drinking it for six to eight days and [he will improve]. (*BAM* 7 37 ii 14′–18′)

These recipes, although exceptional, indicate both specific measured amounts and dosage of medication. Nothing comparable exists within incantation texts or their accompanying rituals. Furthermore, even when no amounts are recorded in medical texts, it was likely that the recipe itself was only a mnemonic and that many of the details regarding how to administer drugs were instructed orally rather than being written down.[29]

There are some important distinguishing patterns of drug application for various ailments. For instance, eye-disease texts use more salves and ointments than drugs taken internally. Although one cannot assume that such general patterns reflect intuitive or rational thinking, they nevertheless show that recipes were designed specifically for specific ailments and that relatively few recipes were panaceas, used for any and all ailments.[30]

Some recipes may have been widely used because of some desired medicinal effect deemed to be useful for more than one condition. We are not referring here to any modern notions of side-effects or medical properties, but rather to what might have been perceived by ancient physicians as medically relevant. Many parts of the human body, for instance, were examined to see if they were hard or soft, or wet or dry, and drugs or diet could be administered in order to correct any abnormal condition, since this was considered to have serious consequences on general health. For example, drugs thought capable of drying a patient's loose stools (which were "wet") might also be thought effective in drying up a "wet" cough (which produced excessive sputum or phlegm).[31] Our ability to assess these conditions is severely hampered by our inability to identify ancient Babylonian plant and mineral names and hence drugs, in order to assess any chemical properties behind Babylonian prescriptions.

Types of disease classifications in medical texts differ from each other significantly. "Kidney-disease" and "rectal disease" were, transparently, seated in specific *organs*. The designation *suālu* or "cough" for a type of disease refers to a *symptom* of the illness, while Hand of the Ghost refers to a potential *cause* of the disease (in theory, at least). Given that there were many facets to the Babylonian disease repertoire, it is unclear why very different conditions were often treated with the same prescriptions.

Regarding the overall structure and contents of typical medical treatises from Babylonia, the primary information comes from rubrics on medical texts themselves, which are intended to label the contents of the recipes, according to the conditions being treated (see Attinger 2008: 26f.). Typical rubrics are as follows: "if a man's teeth are 'ill'," "if a man's eyes are 'ill'," "if a man's 'heart' (e.g. bowels) is ill," "if a man's breathing is labored (lit. heavy)," "if a man suffers from paralysis (*šaššaṭu*)." Other rubrics offer a bit more relevant information, such as, "if a man suffers from cough, turning into colic,"[32] "if a man's neck sinews hurt, it is the Hand of a Ghost," or simply medical conditions generally ascribed to the Hand of a Ghost (Scurlock 2006: 5–20). One important series is more comprehensive than others, "if a man's brain (*muhhu*)[33] contains heat," which mostly concerns fever in the body.[34] Migraine is referred to as a disease affecting the temples, which corresponds to numerous incantations for headache within the magic corpus. Rubrics, however, do not always explain the nature of the disease, e.g. one set of recipes organized under the heading, "if a man suffers prematurely from groin pain" (Geller 2005: 102f.). Finally, we also find medical texts with rubrics that are clearly magical in nature, labeling recipes as belonging to a category of $uš_{11}$-búr-ru-da, "breaking the spell" or zi-ku_5-ru-da, "cutting the breath,"[35] which are well known in otherwise magical contexts.

These rubrics do not, however, exhaust the full range of diseases which Babylonian medical texts aimed to treat. Aside from ailments just mentioned, medical texts dealt with diseases specifically associated with a certain part of the anatomy, such as kidney disease, rectal disease, diseases of the lung and chest, gall bladder disease, and many kinds of skin ailments, diseases of the foot and tendon, and diseases affecting the mouth and nose which resemble some aspects of leprosy. Other diseases are more general, such as stroke and seizures, which would probably include forms of epilepsy. Baldness was considered to be a treatable disease (or at least one for which we have recipes). Various kinds of fevers and paralysis are medicated, as are digestive problems and general internal disorders, probably occurring almost anywhere in the abdomen. Childbirth was, in some sense, treated as a medical problem. The designations and classification of diseases is not very different from what we find in the Hippocratic corpus, although in almost no instance can we expect to give a modern diagnosis based upon symptoms described in our ancient medical literature. One good example of this phenomenon is kidney disease caused by hypertension, for which the various symptoms and signs are not located in the kidneys (see George 2002), or venereal disease, which is known as the great imposter since it copies the symptoms of other ailments.

At times medical texts provide clues to causes of diseases, and these often differ from the kinds of causes which are found within incantations (such as demons and vengeful gods). A good example of a disease cause is the eating of hexed foodstuffs causing digestive problems; in medical texts, it is not the hex itself which is the problem but rather the ingesting of food which has been cursed or magically altered.

Sumerian and Akkadian Therapeutic Magic

We must turn to other "sciences" as well, including magic. The oldest surviving types of magical texts come from the mid-third millennium BC, but these early texts are too rudimentary to allow much scope for analysis (see Cunningham 1997: 5–43). The next important phase of magical texts is found in Nippur, towards the end of the third millennium BC, this time in Sumerian only, and the same workshop in Nippur appears to have produced the one complete Sumerian medical text which has survived from antiquity (van Dijk and Geller 2003; Civil 1960). These Sumerian incantations address medical problems, such as headache, along with many other types of catastrophic situations occasioned by the attack of demons, such as the interference with natural husbandry and even the malfunction of musical instruments (Krispijn 2008). The basic understanding of these early texts was that demons were capable of destroying all aspects of the world's natural order.[36]

By the time we arrive at the great Sumerian scribal libraries of the Old Babylonian period, contemporary with Hammurabi, the literary text genres have developed considerably, and Sumerian incantations have become long and complex compositions; the process of translating these texts into Akkadian is beginning. By the first millennium BC these same incantations recur in bilingual Sumerian-Akkadian form, preserved in numerous copies in all major libraries in Mesopotamia.

The incantations are formal and formulaic, usually consisting of a dialogue between Ea and Marduk in their roles as father and son, and also in their roles as God of Wisdom and Divine Exorcist. Marduk observes what is wrong with the patient or victim, reports back to Ea seeking advice about how to help, and after a brief discussion Ea tells Marduk what he needs to know. The ritual instructions, which follow as a separate section, usually (but not invariably) derive from Ea's advice, which confers legitimacy upon the exorcist's activities. There are, on the other hand, other types of formal literary incantations from Mesopotamia, mostly in Akkadian, which mainly deal with protection against witches and witchcraft. There is a third genre of more "down-to-earth" types of magic, concerned with the seamy side of life, such as rivalry at court or love magic, and these incantations are often somewhat more vulgar, both in content and language. This scheme is very skeletal but gives a rough idea of genres.

The essential formal elements of these incantations thus consist of a ritual solution to the patient's difficulties being communicated via a dialogue between Marduk and his father Ea. This dialogue becomes so integral to Mesopotamian magic that it is even repeated later on within Akkadian incantations, even when there is no Sumerian original source.[37] Here is an atypical example of the dialogue, with slightly different *dramatis personae*:

> Girra approached Marduk and spoke to him of this
> and in the quiet of his couch at night, (Marduk) listened to this matter.
> (Marduk) entered the temple, to his father Ea, and called out,
> "My father, Girra has approached the East, and news of them has reached (here).
> Hasten to learn the ways of the Seven, and seek out their places."
> "Wise son of Eridu,"
> Ea answered his son Marduk.
> "My son, the Seven among them dwell in the Netherworld,
> and have come here from the Netherworld.
> The Seven were born in the Netherworld,
> and were reared in the Netherworld.
> They have approached here to tread on the edge of the Apsû.
> Go, my son Marduk:
> As for the *e'ru*-wood sceptre of the (protective) spirits (*rābiṣu*),
> in the middle of which Ea is invoked by name,
> and along with the august Eridu incantation formula of purification,
> apply fire to the tip and base (of the sceptre), so that the Seven of them do not draw near to the patient.
> Toss (the flame) like a broad net spread out in a broad place,
> so that it may constantly be present at his head at high noon, and both day and night.
> Let (the sceptre) be held in his hand to light up the street and thoroughfare at night.
> let (the sceptre) be present at the head of the distraught man in the middle of the night,
> (even) during normal sleep in bed." (Utukkū Lemnūtu 13–15: 61–81 [Geller 2007c: 244f.])

This dialogue has a calculated function within the context of the incantation. The officiating exorcist can claim that his incantation comes directly from the gods and that the patient is benefiting from the best possible magic available. Later Akkadian incantations adopt a similar strategy within other contexts, in which the exorcist declares that "the incantation is not mine," and that the spell comes directly from the gods. Nothing therefore depends upon the exorcist's own personal charisma. The dialogue between gods was intended to inspire the patient's confidence, since the patient's acceptance and internalizing of the words and ritual procedures becomes part of the healing process. The exorcist, however, was not trying to dupe the patient into accepting a fiction, since he too would have believed in a dialogue between gods in the same way that the patient believed it.

Sumerian and Akkadian bilingual incantations were eventually compiled into formal compositions or canonized texts by the end of the second millennium BC and formed a large part of ancient libraries. For the most part, these texts recognized the harmful attacks of many kinds of demons and recruited the gods against demons and adjured the demons to depart and not come back. Formal magic lays out the rules of engagement, that whimsical gods can send demons against humans for whatever reason, but usually because humans have upset the gods by committing some transgression or violating some taboo. We rarely hear the patient's own voice in describing his difficulties, although his plight is catalogued in detail by the exorcist, who occasionally speaks in the first person. The patient himself, described throughout as a "man son of his god" and as the "distraught man," is the passive object of all that is happening around him, but the incantations are written from the perspective of the exorcist, not the patient.

Other types of incantations take a slightly different view of man's affairs, although probably dating from a later period than bilingual compositions. Dingir.šà.dib.ba (*ilī ul idi*) incantations have the patient declaring that he does not know what he has done wrong (Lambert 1974: 270). These incantations express the patient's own anxieties in the first person and we hear his voice, expressing his fears, worries, or doubts. These types of incantations also include a lengthy confessional, based upon the assumption that the patient is ill or suffering because he violated some divine taboo, willingly or unwittingly (van der Toorn: 1985, 42f.)

Another series of incantations are collected under the title "Šurpû," which means "burning" referring to a specific ritual. Šurpu incantations provide the long confessional of sins, defined as violation of an ancient taboo, and these taboos are delineated within the incantation itself.

Šurpu incantations also have much in common with formal Sumerian-Akkadian bilingual magic, probably originating in the second millennium BC. Tablet IX (equivalent to a "chapter") of Šurpu consists of what are known as *Kultmittelbeschwörungen*, incantations conveying sanctity on all instruments and paraphernalia used in the relevant rituals. The idea is that any cultic tool used in an exorcism needed to be ritually purified by reciting the appropriate incantation (Cunningham 1997: 112f.).

Formal magic also must deal with the attack of ghosts rather than demons, when a restless spirit returns from the other world to attack living humans. The texts give many different reasons for a ghost to re-emerge, usually involving not being buried with the proper funerary rites because the person died at sea or in the steppe, or simply had no living descendants to make the required periodic funerary offerings. Of particular danger was the Ardat Lilî, the Maiden Lilith, who never married or had children and died before having normal sexual relations, and she thus returns to seek out sex with susceptible human partners. The Maiden Lilith is no demon, however; she is a ghost, which means that she was not created by the gods with the expressed purpose of causing harm, but she herself was a victim in her own life and she is looking for compensation among the living. On the other hand, she is potentially as harmful as any demon and incantations are needed against her visitation. Ardat Lilî is usually portrayed as a victim, defended by her patron goddess Ištar:

> The evil demon *took away* the maiden from the palace of the steppe.
> The one who was unnamed from the start pursued her relentlessly.
> The incorporeal one pursued her relentlessly.
> He struck her hand and placed (it) on his (own) hand,
> he struck her foot and placed (it) on his foot,
> he struck her head and placed (it) upon his head.
> She therefore enters the pure *gipar*.
> The woman (=Ištar) shook the heavens and made the earth quake.
> The proud pure Ištar cried out in heaven and earth,
> she burned, she was inflamed, she took an oath at the door of the upper room:
> "The evil Utukku and Alû demons must not enter the house,
> the evil Utukku demon who seized him (the victim) must stand aside,
> but may the good Utukku-spirit and genius be present at his side." (Utukkū Lemnūtu 5 183–95 [Geller 2007c: 213f.])

This notion of the returning ghost was a well-known folk motif in antiquity, and the ritual for getting rid of a maiden lilith also appears in several different Akkadian contexts, for which the most effective ritual appeared to be the use of a marriage between male and female figurines, to attempt to alleviate the maiden ghost's sexual frustrations (Farber 2004: 117–32). Nevertheless, the actual descriptions of the attack of ghosts, like that of demons, is detached from any question regarding the patient's own thoughts or fears. Everything is in the third person.

In the third major type of incantation, Maqlû, we encounter a text of a completely different sort. For one thing, the subject matter concerns witches and witchcraft, not ordinary demons and ghosts. Also, texts appear in the first person, with the patient complaining that the witch attacks *me*, and hence the witch is addressed in the second person.

> Because a witch has bewitched me,
> A deceitful woman has accused me
> Has (thereby) caused my god and goddess to be estranged from me (and)
> I have become sickening in the sight of anyone who beholds me,
> I am therefore unable to rest day and night. (Maqlû I 4–8, translation Abusch 2002: 30)

> I call forth (lit. seek out) against you (O witch) cult-players and ecstatics;
> I (for my part) will break your bond.
> May warlocks bewitch you, I will break your bond.
> May witches bewitch you, I will break your bond.
> May cult-players bewitch you, I will break your bond.
> May ecstatics bewitch you, I will break your bond. (Maqlû VII 92–7, translation Abusch 2002: 10)

At first glance, it seems that we ought to have in Maqlû a more intimate view of the patient in which he expresses his own fears and anxieties, but a more extensive look at the text leaves us in doubt. The text itself is repetitive in places and formulaic, almost like liturgy, and we assume that this lengthy and nicely phrased text was intended to be recited by the patient or by a proxy, such as the incantation priest. So although Maqlû is important for showing an awareness in magical texts of the patient's psychological state, it provides little more than general descriptions of angst, depression, and paranoia.[38]

Incantations, for the most part, address the familiar problems of disease and death threatening the patient, but magic is designed to deal with the more supernatural causes of disease, such as the revenge of an angry god, witchcraft, or the patient's own breaking of ancient taboos and the subsequent forfeiting of any divine protection against demons and disease. By its very nature of dealing with the supernatural (gods, demons, witches), magic is classified lower down on the scale of scientific

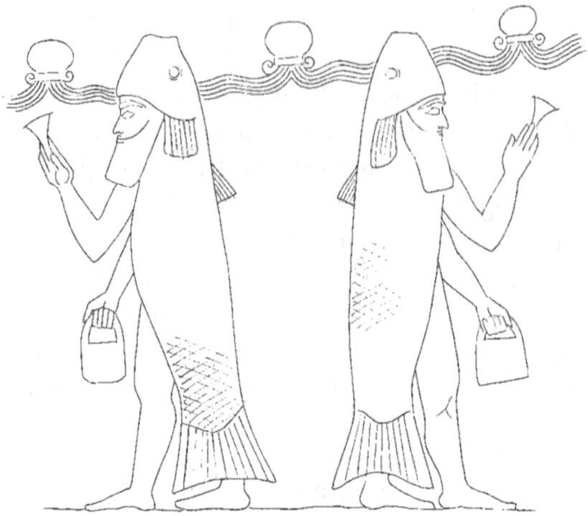

Figure 1.2 Exorcists performing a ritual, dressed as fish-men *apkallu* sages (Vorderasiatisches Museum, Berlin; drawing Tessa Rickards)

texts, bearing in mind our rule based on mathematics as a necessary component of scientific thinking. Magical texts comprised one of the disciplines forming a major part of the school curriculum in Babylon (Gesche 2001: 214f.), and the Babylon tablet libraries contained many varieties of magical texts. Although magical texts were mostly poetic and can be considered important examples of *belles lettres*, at the same time incantations and their associated rituals were designed for very practical purposes of influencing human health and fortunes, and hence represent applied "science." Although the concept of magic itself was to alter the effects of supernatural forces (demonic attacks, curses, even fate), the real effect of such texts was to alter the psychological state of a patient by reducing levels of anxiety and neurotic fear. The "science" of magic is based upon a profound understanding of human psychology grasped by the composers of these incantations and consisted of an impressive repertoire of incantations for very different purposes, aimed at alleviating feelings of guilt, helplessness, paranoia, anger, obsession, or other types of personality disorder. Nevertheless, there is little within magic that can be quantified or measured, and hence magic only merits a rather low score on our scientific quotient.

Examples of magical texts are numerous, and the following incantation tablet from Persian period Nippur in Babylonia (c. 500 BC) is a prayer addressed to the sun god Šamaš and to Gula, goddess of healing, on behalf of a patient whose illness is ascribed either to the attack of demons, or to a worm. It is the alternative of supernatural and natural causes of disease which makes the incantation interesting from the point of view of ancient science:

> Incantation: Šamaš, lord and sublime judge of heaven and earth,
> Nintinugga (Gula), lady who brings the dead back to life,
> who are able to heal kings and servants;
> a man – tired, sleepless, and weary –
> in whose body there is disease, malaria, *lamaštu*-demon(-disease),
> jaundice, *chill*,[39] or parasites,
> which destroy the whole of a man's body;
> by the command of Ea, Šamaš, Marduk,
> and Nintinugga (Gula), may disease go out!
> As for malaria, *lamaštu*-demon(-disease), jaundice, *chill*,
> and parasites which are in his body,
> may they (all) go out and may the man recover.
> Incantation of Damu, Gula, and Dingirmah. Spell. (Nougayrol 1947: 41)

Psychosomatic Illness

The distinctions between *soma* (body) and *psyche* (soul) can be found in the Hippocratic corpus, and the notion of psychosomatic illness can be traced back to Plato, who writes, "When the soul is too strong for the body and of ardent temperament, she dislocates the whole frame and fills it with ailments from within" (*Timaeus*, translation Robinson 2006: 51). Similarly, older parts of the Hippocratic corpus described the diseased mind as exhibiting characteristic types of behavior, which include talking too much or not at all, exhibiting unmotivated or exaggerated moods and emotions, or speaking more aggressively or greeting people more warmly than warranted by the occasion (Gundert 2006: 34f.).

No corresponding conceptual framework can be found in Akkadian, which lacks any term or concept of "soul,"[40] but the distinction between physical and mental illness can be found in Babylonian medicine, although not expressed in the same philosophical form. An example of this phenomenon comes from Babylonian medical texts dealing with anti-witchcraft activities, of which we have a considerable number (Schwemer 2007: 165–79). Tablets dealing with witchcraft, however, differed considerably from anti-witchcraft tablets within the medical corpus. To illustrate the point, here are two examples of medical anti-witchcraft therapy:

> If a man is seized by the "Hand of a Ghost"(-disease), or is seized by "epilepsy" (*bennu*), or is seized by stroke (*antašubbû*),
> Saghulhaza(-disease) has seized him, Lugalurra(-disease) has seized him, "Hand of a God"(-disease) has seized him,
> "Hand of a Goddess"(-disease) has seized him, "Hand of an Oath" (-disease) has seized him, "Hand of Mankind"(-disease) has seized him,
> the Alû-demon has overwhelmed him, insanity ("change of mind") has seized him, he is sick with ague (*himittu*),
> he faces rage, anger, and rejection of god and goddess,
> his ears buzz, he keeps having depression ("broken heart"), he forgets what he says,
> he talks to himself, gets heated, vacillates, can't make up his mind,
> gives an order and changes his mind, he constantly sustains losses,
> fear at night, and all day long he is in a daze,
> he has quarrels at home and brawls in the street, one looks at him with malevolence, he is cursed by many people.
> He swears in his mind to a goddess foolishly.
> This is what that man [the witch] has over him by way of wrath of god and goddess!
> In order to dissolve these (conditions) so that his anxieties not overcome him, and for
> these sicknesses to be removed from his body, [perform the following rituals] ... (Farber 1977: 56, 64; see Stol 1999: 65)

> If a man's limbs tremble like (those of) a sick man,
> ... his feet and his *stomach-lining* are slack,
> he speaks but nothing comes out,
> he is robbed of his potency (lit. erection), his mood is always bad,
> whether when urinating or
> when he sleeps with a woman his semen is ejaculated (prematurely),
> that man is not pure, god and goddess turn him away,
> his command is not obeyed. (Farber 1977: 227, 237)

The texts above assume the format of medical rather than magical texts. Instead of the usual notations for magical spells, these passages both begin with the standard diagnostic phrase typical of medical texts, "if a man (suffers from) ...". This formal distinction between magical and medical tablets from Mesopotamia is a fixed tradition which is not subject to alteration, and the diagnostic format of the passages above should technically be classified as medical. On the other hand, the rituals which accompany these medical-like diagnostic descriptions of mental illnesses are more magical than medical. The first ritual (see Farber 1977: 56, 64) involves bringing an offering of ash-baked cakes to a shepherd, which is used to purchase a virgin kid. The next step is to sweep and wash the roof of the house and set up an altar to the goddess Gula, on which various offerings and libations are made (dates, flour, honey, butter, beer, and breads), with incense being burned. Some strands of the client's hair and garment hem are weighed in a balance in the presence of a chanting priest. The kid is then sacrificed and skinned, and the client recites an incantation. A similar ritual is performed for the second passage above (Farber 1977: 227, 237) in which the client is thoroughly purified over several days, an altar with foodstuffs is set up for Ištar and Dumuzi, and a sheep is sacrificed. On this occasion male and female figurines with arms being bound behind the back are constructed out of various materials (clay, gypsum, dough, fat), and appropriate incantations are recited.

A comparable case is described in the following medical text describing depression, for which the ritual prescribes a formal marriage ceremony between a male and female figurine, accompanied by offerings and the sacrifice of a sheep.

> If a man suffered a mishap but he did not know what had happened to him, he was constantly having regular reverses and losses, losses of barley and of money [...], (or) losses of male and female servants, oxen, horses or flocks, dogs, and pigs, and even people were dying all at once: he kept having depression ("broken heart"). When he spoke, no one listened, and calling there was no answer. Taking people's complaints to heart, he lies frightened in his bed. He has paralysis. No holy water has come near him, and he is fed up with god and king. His limbs are flaccid and he gets increasingly afraid, not sleeping night and day and having terrifying dreams. He keeps having paralysis. He has less bread and beer (and) he forgets what he says. That man has earned the anger of god and goddess upon him, his own personal god and goddess are upset with him. If that man suffers from the Hand of the Oath, Hand of the God, Hand of Mankind or suffers from moaning, or the guilt of father, mother, sister or brother family, relations, and kin has affected him, in order to resolve it so that his worries (i.e. melancholy) do not overwhelm [him]: (Ritual follows). (*BAM* 234; see Ritter and Kinnier Wilson 1980: 24–27)[41]

Although the text does not specify why a ritual marriage is required, we can presume that the client's mental anguish is determined as being caused by the amorous intentions of a maiden lilith (*ardat lilî*), a feared succubus, and that the purpose of the marriage was to provide a spouse to address her sexual needs. In other cases, a similar diagnosis of mental imbalance was attributed to sorcery (Stol 1999: 67). Although these texts are all examples of the grey area between medicine and magic, other medical texts dealing with mental problems resort to more traditional kinds of recipes for dealing with the symptoms. A good example of this can be found in a late Uruk medical text from the third century BC, which deals with anxiety and depression (von Weiher 1983: No. 22; von Weiher 1988: No. 85).[42] The patient imagines that he has a rival or enemy who causes him to experience hatred, perversions of justice, loss of breath, and aphasia when faced with authority (god or king), he suffers from anxiety day and night and in his dreams imagines himself to be the object of constant slander and gossip. The remedy for this poor mental state is various herbs and minerals being wrapped in a leather pouch to be hung from his neck. Although the prescription might appear more magical than medical to us, in ancient terms the use of drugs wrapped in a leather pouch was a standard medical procedure, seen to be more directly curative (like a potion) than like an amulet (see Farber 1973). A similar text (*BAM* 316) reads as follows:

> If a man is constantly frightened and worries day and night; losses are suffered regularly by him and his profit is cut off; people speak defamation about him, his interlocutor does not speak affirmatively, a finger of derision is stretched out (i.e. pointed) after him; in the palace where he appears he is not well received; his dreams are confused, in his dreams he keeps seeing dead people; heartbreak is laid upon him; the wrath of god and goddess is upon him, god and goddess are angry with him; witchcraft has been practiced against him; he has been cursed before god and goddess; his omens are confused; (city) god, king, noble, and prince are annoyed with him; as many as seven times his case (lit. judgment) is not cleared up (lit. is not straight[ened out]) by diviner or dream interpreter; he is beset by speaking but not being heard (and responded to favourably). (Translation Abusch 2002: 31–2)

There is no doubt about the genre of this text, since it occurs within a medical prescription. The ritual (not translated by Abusch) is revealing about how Babylonian physicians dealt with this kind of psychological trauma:

> Its ritual: you wrap in (a) leather (bag) *taramuš, imhur-lim, imhur-ešra, erkulla, elkulla, amēlānu*(-plants),

coral, tamarisk, (and) "mace"-plant;
recite over him seven times the incantation *alah salah bašinti*
(and) the incantation *arazu šutemab*[43] and place (the bag) [on] his neck.

Like in the previous case of amulet stones and incantations being prescribed for psychological distress, this ritual calls for medicinal plants and drugs to be hung around the patient's neck, along with appropriate incantations being recited.[44] In both cases, medicinal plants and amuletic stones hanging on the patient's body are often used with somatic illnesses, which may show that these types of mental conditions resemble illnesses in which physical symptoms are attributable to psychic causes.

The magical corpus was also designed to deal with a patient's anxieties, to help him recognize the hidden and harmful forces of the surrounding cosmos, to acknowledge the ultimate causes for misfortune and ill-health, and to try to reconcile the patient with whatever is acting against him. Mesopotamian man was full of fear of transgression, for which there were abundant opportunities, such as eating the wrong foods on the wrong day, or having intercourse with an unclean (menstruating) woman. Essentially, while magic intended to explore the ultimate causes of illness and misfortune, it employed a variety of strategies to reverse the processes. In some cases, the patient was asked to make his confession from a long list of sins (Šurpu Tablet II), while in other cases the magic threatened retribution and revenge against demons and purveyors of evil, such as malevolent witches (Schwemer 2007: 143). Other types of magic include curses against rivals and enemies, which are relatively less common, possibly because they originally represent a type of folk magic which belonged to oral tradition or in later times was more common in Aramaic. There are even cases of love incantations within Mesopotamian magic, in which black magic is employed to force a woman to abandon her family and run off with the subject of the incantation, but this type of incantation can be seen within the context of unrequited love as a type of sickness, for which the incantation serves as a means of relief from psychic torment (Geller 2003). Other kinds of incantations deal with fear of ghosts, bad dreams, sex with a succubus, or against dog-bite and snakebite, all of which intend to offer the patient some kind of relief against real or imagined harms. We have no incantations, on the other hand, specifically designated to treat depression or obsessive-compulsive behavior, although Babylonian therapists had enough grasp of human psychology to recognize these disorders, and it is likely that magic was employed to deal with such problems in an indirect way.

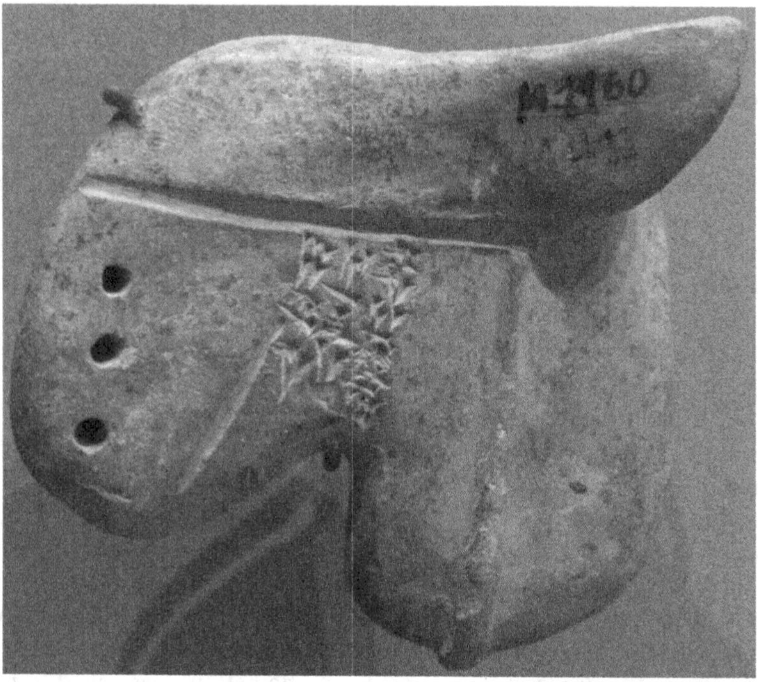

Figure 1.3 Clay model of a sheep liver used for divination, from Mari in Syria, second millennium BC (Musée du Louvre; photo Florentina Badalanova Geller)

Magic could be summarized as expressions of anxiety and worry about angry gods, malicious demons, harmful witches. There is another level on which to understand magic, as expressions of human psychology without reference to the actual existence (or not) of gods, demons, and witches. The relationship between humans and gods, as expressed in prayers and religious literature, is that of child to parent or of servant to master, and a child's fear of punishment for misbehavior reflects a similar pattern of fear between humans and gods. Divine anger and punishment was thought to apply even when human transgression was committed unintentionally; the essential relationship between man and god in Mesopotamia was that of fear. Incantations expressing the patient's alarm at being the object of divine wrath are understandable within these terms. Nevertheless, it is difficult to ascertain from this literature when any particular patient exceeded the boundaries of normal fear of gods and became excessively anxious, or in modern terms, neurotic.

We are also faced with a perverse sort of logic within magic, namely that if a person is ill or suffers misfortune, then this is *a priori* evidence that the gods are angry with him. This argument is less a matter of anxiety and more a way of explaining the cause of illness in a way one could easily grasp: the gods are ultimately responsible for human fate and they are angry. Appease the gods and reduce the chances of further illness or misfortune.

Divination

Omens formed one of the most important parts of Babylon's school curriculum (Gesche 2001; Cryer 1994: 139–40). In some ways, divination can be classified as the least "scientific" among Babylon's disciplines, since the entire concept of divination is based upon the logical fallacy that two events in sequence are thought of as being causally related. Hence, the entrails of a sheep with a specific characteristic were thought to forecast some significant contemporary events, usually affairs of state. Nevertheless, the result of this logical fallacy had certain fortuitous consequences as far as scientific thinking is concerned: the ancient divination scholars collected large databases of ominous events (also from positions of celestial objects, flights of birds, patterns of oil on water or smoke, unnatural births, and many other genres of omens). The practice of collecting and sorting data, as well as analyzing data, must be seen as a process resembling certain aspects of scientific thinking. So although the aims of divination can be seen as heading off on the wrong tack, the methods and procedures of handling data, and the idea of drawing inferences from large amounts of data, should be seen as a type of forerunner to modern science.

In this way, the position of constellations or planets, or the sun or moon (e.g. eclipses) within the heavens was considered to be relevant to events happening on earth. It is difficult to know which discipline came first, astronomy or astrology. Was careful observation of heavenly bodies later applied to celestial divination, or did the "science" relating movements in the night sky to events on earth become the basis for astronomy? Whatever the rationale for watching the heavens, astrology by the Persian and later Hellenistic periods was flourishing and developed horoscopes which later influenced Greek thought, later to become the common pseudo-science of every newspaper in the modern world.

As for medical omens and the relationship between divination and medicine, the Diagnostic Handbook preserves its own unique style, which differs significantly from the way diseases and symptoms are usually described in therapeutic recipes (see Fincke 2006–7: 144f.;

Stol 1991–2: 64f.). While therapeutic recipes open with an "if" clause defining the symptoms, they are not casuistic in the same way that legal or omen texts operate. "If" the patient suffers from a certain disease or syndrome or ailment, the recipes provide instructions regarding what to do "in order to cure him," and as a result "he will get better" or "he will improve"; the conclusion is always positive. This differs fundamentally from the Diagnostic Handbook, which maintains the classical structure of omen texts, i.e. if such-and-such, then such-and-such (may result). In most cases the result will be that the patient will die, that his illness will be prolonged, or that he might survive and improve, and variations of these possibilities are given within a limited range of possibilities.

The search for parallels to the Diagnostic Handbook outside the genre of medical literature takes us to a group of first-millennium BC commentaries which were primarily academic in origin, known as *Multābiltu*-omens (Koch 2005). This group consists primarily of highly specialized explanatory texts on liver divination, and the texts provide general guidelines for interpreting omens and omen texts, based upon specific rules of exegesis. Hence, the concept of "long" implies "success," so that if a certain key physiological feature of an examined liver is "long," this portends that the king will have success in battle (see Jeyes 1980: 23f.). However, to proceed correctly one must know whether a "long" part of the liver anatomy is associated with the right or left half of the liver, since "long" on the left side may mean that it is one's enemy who has success.[45] This unusual divination text is highly theoretical and may reflect oral tradition (George 2008: 557) or discussions within the academy, as do other types of commentaries.

It must be emphasized that *Multābiltu*-omens belong squarely to divination and not medicine, despite the fact that an entire tablet (i.e. chapter) is devoted to omens taken on behalf of a patient. The seventh tablet begins with the phrase, "if you perform an examination of the liver (*têrtu*) for the well-being of the patient …" (Koch 2005: 154). What follows is a series of technical omens referring to an animal liver, with a typical protasis (or "if"-clause) as follows: "if you perform an extispicy (liver examination) and there are two 'paths' to the right of the gall bladder and two 'paths' to the left of the gall bladder …". Then comes the actual prediction, most commonly, "the patient will die" (Koch 2005: 155: 13′, 158, 560), but there are variations on this theme, such as, "the calmed patient who ate food and drank water will [have a relapse] of his illness [and die]," or the patient "will change his residence and get well" (Koch 2005: 155, 12–14). Occasionally the patient will contract a disease but then recover or the illness will linger (Koch 2005: 156, 17–18). Such expressions are similar to those found in the Diagnostic Handbook.

One telling medical comment found in *Multābiltu* refers to the physician's withdrawing treatment from a patient in cases with a fatal prognosis. The interpretation of one such omen is that "the patient will get worse; depart quietly, do not perform any [treatment]" (Koch 2005: 156, 16).[46] It was not the diviner's task to offer or withhold medical treatment, so we have to presume either that the physician was an interested party to this particular omen, or that the information would be communicated to the physician, if appropriate. In any case, we have little information regarding the use of divination for patients, except for the meager references in the Neo-Assyrian letters and diviners' reports.

Other omen hermeneutics resemble diagnostic omens, such as diseases being labeled as the Hand of (a certain) God, and in *Multābiltu* Tablet VII we indeed find the "Hand of Marduk," "Hand of Ištar," as well as the "Curse of Ea," all designations of disease. One particularly revealing omen stipulates:

> If, ditto [= you perform the divination], and you perform (it) for the "Hand of a God," the patient will live until his appointed time, but after his appointed time he will die. (Koch 2005: 155, 13)

This omen is inserted out of sequence with the rest of the omens, which usually refer to an anatomical feature in the animal's liver, but uniquely not here. Obviously, the problem was to determine whether the disease was indeed caused by the "Hand of the God," or to determine precisely which god had brought the disease. In any case, this omen is predictive and not therapeutic, and the result will be that the patient will live or die according to his destiny decided by the gods.

The similarities between the omen apodoses of *Multābiltu* and the apodoses of the Diagnostic Handbook are unmistakable, and there seems to be only one inference to be drawn, that these texts derive from the same scribal source. On the surface, this conflicts with the supposition that omen divination was composed and copied by diviners[47] while diagnostic omens by exorcists. In fact, the authorship of these texts is more complicated. It is probably true that in the second millennium BC discrete genres of texts were composed by the professionals who actually used the texts, so that incantations were composed by exorcists and divination texts by diviners, etc. By the time of Assurbanipal's great library, however, the situation has already changed. No less than five *Multābiltu* texts found in Nineveh were copied by the renowned scholar

Nabû-zuqup-kēna in 711 BC (Koch 2005: 267). Although Nabû-zuqup-kēna refers to himself as *ṭupšarru*, "scribe," his wide knowledge and the impressive range of texts he copied show him to be a master of cuneiform literature. Certainly not a diviner, he took an interest in academic divination texts, such as those found in the *Multābiltu* corpus.

So although these large compendia of scientific texts found in Nineveh or Assur libraries go back to earlier prototypes from the second millennium BC, it seems likely that strict lines separating the professionals from one another was steadily breaking down in the first millennium (see Parpola 1983: 8). One of the *Multābiltu* texts found in the late Uruk library was copied by the prolific scribe and *mašmaššu*-exorcist Iqīšâ (Koch 2005: 209), who had a vast repertoire of tablets under his belt, including scholarly commentaries.

Since the Diagnostic Handbook was arguably the original (or older) composition upon which *Multābiltu* Tablet VII was modeled, this would tell us little about the milieu in which the Diagnostic Handbook itself was composed. It is true that the Diagnostic Handbook is attested already in the Old Babylonian period, from about 1700 BC. Nevertheless, the rapid growth of scholarship during the first millennium produced a much broader range of texts than had been known earlier, and it is likely that scientific literature grew up within the academy as schools became more widespread and specialized. It is also highly probable that the Diagnostic Handbook, like *Multābiltu*, was essentially a scholarly or theoretical composition, used to teach the theory of diagnosis, rather than a vade mecum which the doctor would carry with him to the patient's bedside, to look up the appropriate symptoms while examining the patient. It is quite possible, in fact, that the Diagnostic Handbook was never actually used by practicing physicians, but was a speculative treatise on diagnosis, much as we might find in the Hippocratic corpus or in Aristotle. The therapeutic recipes, on the other hand, probably existed in small single-tablet formats that may have actually represented prescriptions from the practice of medicine, and these were later copied into the great library and medical archives which we find in Nineveh, Assur, Babylon, Uruk, and other sites.

2

Who Did What to Whom?

As we have seen, Babylonian healing therapy was divided between the activities of the *mašmaššu*-exorcist and the *asû*-"physician," each operating within his own area of expertise, although not in a way intuitively obvious to modern medical practitioners. According to Paul-Alain Beaulieu, in later periods "prevention and cure, spiritual as well as physical, were both placed under the care of the exorcist" (Beaulieu 2007: 479). The exorcist was responsible for magical prevention of attacks of demons, angry gods, or even witchcraft and unfavorable omens, and he could also act as attending physician who visited the patient on his sick bed to give a prognosis, predicting the nature and course of the disease (see below). The exorcist had all the social advantages of being a priest. The *asû*-physician, on the other hand, appeared to have acted more as an apothecary who prepared the complicated recipes and drugs. As a layman, he had no access to the temple and presumably operated from a corner shop in the street or from his home. The exorcist operated primarily under the assumption that disease was ultimately caused by divine will or fate; the *asû*, while generally agreeing with this position, concentrated more on natural causes of symptoms (bites, excessive exposure to draughts or sunlight, kidney stone, etc.).

In order to better understand the respective roles of exorcist and physician, it may help to delve into some basic terminology. There are two different terms for "exorcist" in Akkadian, and many in Sumerian. The Akkadian term *āšipu*, a more literary term for exorcist, refers to the professional priest who mastered the "art of exorcism," *āšipūtu*. These terms are difficult to etymologize since the cognate verb *wašāpu* "to exorcise" is probably derived from the noun and probably only denotes that which the *āšipu* was supposed to do (i.e. perform exorcisms); the circular logic tells us little (see Cavigneaux 1999: 254f.; *pace* Jean 2006: 19f.); Aramaic, Mandaic, and Syriac cognates are likely to be derived from Akkadian. The other word for "exorcist," *mašmaššu*, was the most commonly used term within private letters and colophons of tablets, and since this term is much more widely attested in documents than *āšipu*, it is the term for exorcist which we prefer.[48] Unlike *āšipu*, it is a word we can attempt to etymologize.

The word *mašmaššu* may derive from a root *mašāšu*, "to wipe," with the Sumerian word and logogram maš.maš possibly being a Semitic loanword. A similar pattern occurs with the Akkadian word *kaškaššu*, "overwhelming," derived from the root *kašāšu*, "to overpower." The term *mašāšu* "to wipe" is not a medical term, nor is it related to *muššu'u*, "to rub or massage," which is genuine medical terminology. On the other hand, "wiping" is one of the key types of ritual acts, as we know from Šurpu incantations (see above) which prescribe wiping the patient down with flour to remove his sins.[49] The original meaning of maš.maš/*mašmaššu* may have originally derived from a term for physiotherapist, only later becoming identified as an exorcist.

An explanation of the meanings behind these professional offices deserves fuller elaboration. For a long time we thought we knew the difference between *āšipu* and *asû*, as expounded in the famous article by Edith Ritter (Ritter 1965). The *āšipu*, we were told, dealt with *āšipūtu* "exorcism"; and handled all matters of magic. The *asû* employed *asûtu* "healing arts" and acted as the doctor. All seemed so very simple.

We now wonder if these magical/medical titles in Mesopotamia are to be taken any more seriously than the title of *Dottore* in *commedia dell'arte*. Revisionists now dominate and we are no longer as certain about the roles of doctors and exorcists, magicians and sorcerers and apothecaries. The extant corpus of medical texts, for instance, contains many examples of medical texts which were either owned or copied by exorcists. Furthermore, it is not clear who actually composed the incantations within the *medical* corpus, since they seem so very different from incantations within formal exorcisms. On the other hand, was it really part of the physician's brief to write spells? The patient's role within this scheme is also unknown, since we never encounter a proper dialogue within Babylonian medical literature in which the patient is formally asked to describe his symptoms. It seems that the therapist was expected to know what was wrong with the patient without having to ask, like a diviner interpreting his signs, or like a good general practitioner or acupuncturist.

Professional Title Classification

One of the hallmarks of Babylonian scholarship was the lexical list, one of the genres of non-administrative documents to appear in the very beginning of writing, even in early archaic pictograph tablets. The lexical lists became a favorite mode of recording data, usually in the form of a list of Sumerian words or a bilingual list of Sumerian words with an Akkadian translation, and in some cases translations into other languages as well. Even many of the Sumerian unilingual lists were probably bilingual, with the Akkadian equivalent words being recited orally within the school curriculum. One of the oldest lists in the Sumerian lexical corpus is a list of "professions," with early antecedents going back to the third millennium BC, although late versions of this list also include a group of Sumerian designations for "exorcist." The following is a "non-canonical" excerpt from the professional list:

[maš]-maš	= *maš-ma-šu*	"exorcist"
tígi	= *a-ši-pu*	"exorcist" (lit. harpist)
ka-pirig	= MIN (ditto)	"exorcist"
muš-DU$^{\text{la-la-ah}}$DU	= *muš-la-la-ah-hu*	"snake-charmer"
lú-^{giš}gàm-šu-du$_7$	= *muš-ši-pu*	"exorcist"
		(MSL 11 102: 204–8)

Items on this list of exorcists are all synonyms for the *mašmaššu* (not *āšipu*), and as such include the snake-charmer and harpist, as well as a rare word for exorcist, *muššipu*, who carries a curved staff, mentioned once only in the standard magical compositions (Šurpu VIII 41). According to this excerpt, *mašmaššu* is not identical with *āšipu*, but a synonym.

Another listing of exorcists is "canonical" and more complete, with more information regarding synonyms for *āšipu*:

[tígi]	= *a-š*[*i-p*]*u*	"exorcist"	
[l]ú-tu$_6$-gál	= KI.MIN (ditto)	"exorcist"	(lit. man having a spell)
ka^{ka}-tu$_6$-gál	= KI.MIN (ditto)	"exorcist"	(lit. mouth having a spell)
ka-kù-gál	= KI.MIN (ditto)	"exorcist"	(lit. [one] having a pure mouth)
ka$^{\text{ka-ap-ri-ig}}$pirig	= KI.MIN (ditto)	"exorcist"	(lit. lion-mouth?)
šim-mú	= KI.MIN (ditto)	"exorcist"	(lit. plant-grower)
inim-kù-gál	= KI.MIN (ditto)	"exorcist"	(lit. [one] having a pure word)

$^{\text{ni-ig-ru}}$KAxAD.KÙ	= KI.MIN (ditto)	"exorcist" (lit. snake-charmer)
nigru	= *muš-lah*$_4$	"snake-charmer"
muš-lah$_4$	= KI.MIN (ditto)	"snake-charmer"

(MSL 12 133: 146–55)

This second listing of Sumerian terms for exorcist is varied and somewhat idiosyncratic, with some overlap with the first list above. The first entry is tígi or "harpist," whom we would probably associate more with liturgy than with incantations, and the list ends with the term nigru or "snake charmer," which probably alludes to the substantial corpus of Sumerian and Akkadian incantations for snakebite and dog-bite, etc. (see Finkel 1999; Jean 2006: 184); nevertheless, the job of snake-charmer would hardly describe the exorcist's primary occupation or concern. The lexical list also defines šim.mú or "apothecary" (lit. grower of medicinal plants) as an exorcist, although some would prefer to see the *asû*-physician as an apothecary (Scurlock 1999: 78). So already three of the entries for exorcist appear controversial. The entries lú-tu$_6$-gál, ka^{ka}-tu$_6$-gál, and ka-kù-gál all allude to the common designation for exorcist in Sumerian incantations, lú-mu$_7$-mu$_7$, literally "incantation-man."

The next entry which strikes our attention is ka.pirig, which is glossed as ka-ap-ri-ig, giving us no doubt about the reading of these signs. According to the Diagnostic Handbook, the standard manual of prognosis and diagnosis, it was the ka.pirig who went to the patient's house to take the omens, note the symptoms, diagnose the patient's condition, and make a prognosis; the ka.pirig has no other identifiable role within the medical or magical corpus. The question is what the term actually means. Although we have some representations of priests officiating in lion outfits, probably in magic ritual contexts (Oppenheim 1943: 32), it is unlikely that pirig means "lion" here. Ungnad made the ingenious suggestion that we might have a learned writing for ka.abrig, meaning the "mouth" or "word" of the *abriqqu*-priest, another learned poetic term for an exorcist (Ungnad 1944: 253), although the idea cannot be substantiated by further proof. Whatever the meaning which lies behind the writing, the ka.pirig is identified in these scholastic lexical lists as an exorcist (*āšipu*). On the other hand, the Diagnostic Handbook never refers to the therapist making house calls as either *āšipu* or *mašmaššu*, but only as ^{lú}ka.pirig, which probably indicates something more than an alternative orthography for exorcist.[50]

One late lexical list of professions (actually referring to types of *ummânu* or "professor") was popular in the late scribal school curriculum (Gesche 2001: 130f.); the names are given below with a more precise translation of the Sumerian terms, although each is translated by *āšipu* "exorcist":

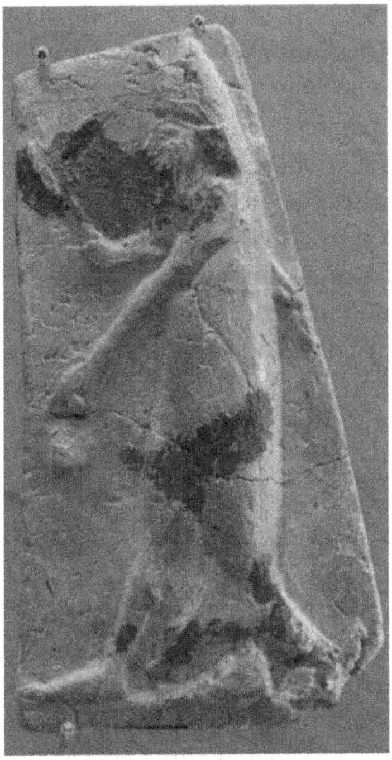

Figure 2.1 Ceramic plaque from the Assyrian period (c. 700 BC) showing an exorcist dressed as an *apkallu* sage (photo Florentina Badalanova Geller)

^{lú}ka.pirig	= *āšipu*	(cf. colophon of the Diagnostic Handbook)
^{lú}ka.luh	= *āšipu*	("mouth-washer")
…		
^{lú}zabar	= *āšipu*	(metalworker)
^{lú}zabar.dab$_5$	= *āšipu*	(functionary)
^{lú}én	= *āšipu*	("incantation-man")
^{lú}maš	= *āšipu*	(see below)
^{lú}maš.maš	= *āšipu*	(*mašmaššu*-exorcist)
^{lú}me	= *āšipu*	(variant of ^{lú}maš)
^{lú}me.me	= *āšipu*	(variant of *mašmaššu*-exorcist)
^{lú}pap.hal	= *āšipu*	("distraught man" = patient)
^{lú}hal	= *āšipu*	(*bārû*-diviner)
^{lú}ad.hal	= *āšipu*	(*bārû*-diviner)
^{lú}pìrig	= *āšipu*	(lion-man)
^{lú}pìrig.tur	= *āšipu*	(leopard-man)

This listing of *āšipu* synonyms affords plenty of surprises.[51] The Sumerian words for exorcist include the one who performs the "mouth-washing" purification ritual (^{lú}ka.luh), as well as the *barû* or diviner (^{lú}hal and ^{lú}ad.hal).[52] The ^{lú}ka.pirig features as well, but we have a new entry, the ^{lú}zabar, the "bronze man," who may have been responsible for making figurines. We even have the ^{lú}pap.hal as exorcist, which is most peculiar. Although pap.hal in this list is elsewhere translated simply as "man," we know this term from numerous occasions in bilingual incantations where it refers to the patient or victim; he is the man who walks about restlessly, with worry and fretting. But in this list, he is an *āšipu*. Everything, in fact, seems to be subsumed under the title of "exorcist," at least in academic contexts of late scribal school curriculum, which supports Beaulieu's observation that exorcism was the most prominent discipline in first-millennium Babylonia (Beaulieu 2007: 477).

The Exorcist in Sumerian Literature

The word maš.maš occurs first within Sumerian literature in a remarkable passage describing a contest featuring one Urgirnunna, a maš.maš who was expert in nam.maš.maš, "magical arts" (Akkadian *mašmaššūtu*). Within this epic account of rivalry between Enmerkar, King of Uruk and Ensuhgiranna, King of Aratta, a fivefold contest ensued between the maš.maš-exorcist Urgirnunna, defending Aratta, and Sagburu, a witch defending Uruk (Black *et al.* 2006: 3–11). The maš.maš-exorcist created various animals *ex nihilo* by throwing something magical into the river; he conjured up a carp, a ewe, a cow, an ibex, and a gazelle, while Sagburru in turn conjured up an eagle, a wolf, a lion, a leopard, and a tiger. Sagburru won. The point is that the Sumerian term maš.maš in this story really means "wonder-worker" and the abstract term nam.maš.maš refers to "wonder-working", having nothing to do with therapy, healing, incantations, or even exorcism. On the other hand, the epic relates that Urgirnunna, the maš.maš-"wonder-worker," resided in the Gipar temple of Aratta, which can only mean that he was a priest. We are left to speculate how the Sumerian word for a wonder-working priest later became a standard term for exorcist and healer.

Mašmaššu or *Āšipu*?

In colophons and in numerous texts from the first millennium BC, the Sumerian logogram (lú.)maš.maš was the most popular title for "exorcist," which often leaves us in some doubt as to whether to use *mašmaššu* or *āšipu* as an Akkadian equivalent for Sumerian maš.maš. There are reasons, however, for suspecting a bipartite division among Babylonian exorcists. The terms *āšipu* and *mašmaššu* tend to be mutually exclusive since we hardly ever find a listing with both titles; we have personnel either described as *āšipu* or described as *mašmaššu*. Among Middle Assyrian professional titles from the late second millennium BC, we find both *āšipu* and the logogram maš.maš (= *mašmaššu*), but not both together; it is either one title or the other (see Jakob 2003: 528f.). Among later first millennium BC lists of wine consignments from Nimrud, we find officials on the wine lists being "diviners," "exorcists," and "physicians" (listed under their respective logograms ^{lú}hal, ^{lú}maš.maš, and ^{lú}a.zu) (Kinnier Wilson 1972: 74). In colophons, very occasionally we find the scribe recorded syllabically as *a-ši-pu*, but far more common is the logogram (lú.)maš.maš (Hunger 1968: 159, 167f.). The "Haus des Beschwörungspriesters" at Assur is really a household of *mašmaššu*-exorcists, which is the term used consistently to describe the owners or writers of the tablets from this house (Pedersén 1986: ii, 45f.). The same pattern appears in Neo-Assyrian letters, which always refer to the exorcist with the Sumerian logogram maš.maš, yet the exorcists are said to practice *āšipūtu* "exorcism."[53] On the other hand, the so-called Exorcist's Manual (a list of incipits of magical and medical texts for scholastic purposes) refers to itself as *mašmaššūtu*, not *āšipūtu* (Jean 2006: 63). Another esoteric text advises that "when you work with plants, stones, and trees, or *mašmaššūtu*, use its commentary" (Reiner 1995: 130). Is this simply the same as *āšipūtu*?

We have some nagging doubts. Although many different types of activities are included within a general category of *mašmaššūtu* or *āšipūtu*, we may be dealing with sub-specialties. As we have already seen, there is the particular label ka.pirig for the therapist who actually diagnoses the patient, never the *āšipu* or *mašmaššu*. Another category of exorcist may have been the šim.mú, the "plant-grower," or apothecary. There may be other categories which need further investigation, such as the exorcist who specializes in performing the ka.luh (*mīs pî*), the cultic "mouth-washing" rituals (Shibata 2008), or the exorcist who performs Namburbî rituals (Caplice 1967).

But what was the *mašmaššu* if not an *āšipu*?[54] In fact, the traditional translation of "exorcist" for *āšipu*/*mašmaššu* is somewhat restrictive. What he does is usually more than simply perform "exorcism"; the exorcist was responsible for an entire range of rituals, in addition to the occasional exorcism.[55] One difference does appear to emerge within the patterns of our evidence, that *āšipu* may have been a prestige term of scholarship and literature while *mašmaššu* comes from the actual parlance of practice and everyday life.

Priest vs Layman

The exorcist was a priest,[56] while the *asû*-"physician" was a layman and entrepreneur. This difference is of crucial importance in understanding how healing was delivered. Individuals described as exorcists functioned as priests in the temple and also held appointments at court.[57] We do not actually know whether the exorcist was a priest who acted as an exorcist or an exorcist who acted as a priest; we do know that his role became increasingly important within the temples in later periods and by the Hellenistic period "exorcistic arts" (*mašmaššūtu*) dominated the school curriculum, which was mostly confined to temples (Beaulieu 2006: 202). The exorcist was supported by prebends, a share of the temple income, although he was probably entitled to private income as well. But what about the *asû*? We have evidence for *āšipūtu*-prebends, but no evidence for *asû* prebends in administrative records.[58] For one thing, this suggests that the *asû* could not enter the inner temple precincts. The late Akkadian term for a priest in general was *ērib bīti*, "one who could enter the temple," which left the *asû* out. It is also perturbing that the *asû* more or less vanishes from our records by Late Babylonian times, in the latter half of the first century BC.

This is pretty much as things should be; we expect the exorcist to be a priest, since his incantations derive their power and authority from his personal relationship to the gods of incantations, usually Ea and Marduk. The *asû*, on the other hand, has his own relationship with Gula, goddess of healing, but his primary task is not related to the cult. In broadest terms, one goes to the exorcist if one needs a *namburbî*-ritual to undo a bad omen (see Caplice 1967), but one goes to the *asû*-physician if one has a nosebleed. Between these two poles is a full range of various options to choose from.

As a trained craftsman and entrepreneur, the *asû* has something in common with another important figure of Babylonian intellectual circles, the *bārû* "diviner," who was also not a priest, as far as we can tell.[59] The *bārû* was responsible for predictions about the future (mostly affecting the king and nation) based upon examining the entrails of animals, usually rams, and this type of divination was known as *bārûtu*. This particular type of divination is attested in both second and first millennia, although it seems to have faded away as a profession after about 500 BC in favor of the priest-astrologer-scribe whose predictions were based upon observations of movements of stars and constellations.[60] Like the *asû*, there is no record of any *bārûtu* prebends, although it is conceivable that the *bārû* as a freelance specialist could offer his services to the temple (for payment) as well as to a private individual (including the king).[61]

There is one further important difference between *asû*, *bārû*, and *mašmaššu*: the former two could travel wherever they wished, while the *mašmaššu*-exorcist did not normally travel but was attached to the temple or palace. This distinction has consequences which can be traced in our sources. When the Hittite king wishes to invite an expert in healing from Babylonia, he invites a Babylonian *asû*-physician, not an exorcist, and he also invites Egyptian physicians (Burde 1974: 5, 6 n. 15). Mari letters speak of an *asû* coming from another city, Mardamân. In the parody of the Poor Man of Nippur or the Isin physician (see below), the *asû* travels from one place to another to ply his trade. In Hittite, the Sumerian logogram for physician in Mesopotamia, lú.a.zu, was borrowed into Hittite script and used to designate the primary healing professional, who acted as magician as well as doctor; he performed rituals as well as checking oracles (Burde 1974: 9).

What actually happened when patients met a healer, and where did this meeting take place? We do not know if the *asû*-physician ever met a patient, except for the occasional reference in the royal correspondence to a court physician visiting his patient. Unlike the exorcist, we cannot place the *asû* in any designated healing location. Although the temple of Gula (the patron goddess of healing and the *asû*) has been suggested as a possible healing venue (Avalos 1998: 114–28), this is hardly possible since the *asû* was not a priest. So where did he practice? Probably on the street, sitting on his rug and dispensing drugs. This might explain why the *asû* evaporates from Late Babylonian and Seleucid period archives. He was a private healer offering his services for money, and probably not very much money: we have no records of any of his private transactions because most late records are from temple archives or from large family businesses, like that of the Murašu or Egibi families (see Wunsch 2007: 238f.). Small transactions tended not to be recorded, in the same way that one never keeps a receipt from the shoemaker. The *asû* has simply dropped out of sight.

Nor does the *asû* appear to use any designated surgery or treatment centre, such as the reed-hut or *šutukku* associated with the magic rituals, magic circles, and incantations belonging to exorcism (see Figure 2.2). What about the sick person's own house? Could the *asû* have made house calls? Here again, the texts tell us otherwise. The Diagnostic

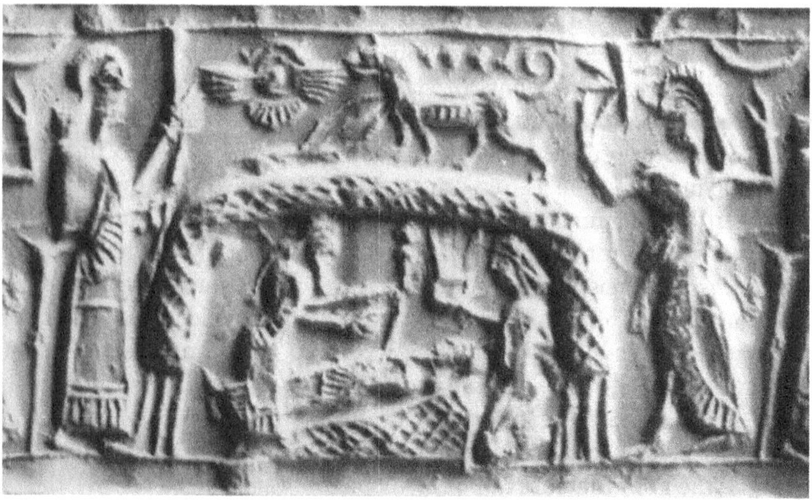

Figure 2.2 Exorcism ritual carried out in a reed *šutukku*-hut, with one woman fumigating and another wailing; early first millennium BC (Collon 1987: No. 803; photo courtesy D. Collon)

Handbook specifically says that it was the ka.pirig-exorcist who visited the patient at home, and not the *asû*. The *asû*-physician may have been an apothecary, a herbalist, even a perfumer, but he had no need of a bedside manner, if we are correctly informed by our texts. It was the exorcist and not the physician who examined the patient from head to foot and recorded the symptoms, and it was the exorcist who needed to have an extensive knowledge of medicine in order to be able to do so. Yet there is a final irony to this story. It was the *asû* who actually won out in the end. The *asû* survived in Aramaic literature, in the form of the *asya*, the doctor, and Aramaic magic bowls offer *asuta* as the main benefit of their magical spells, while after the demise of Akkadian, the *āšipu* and *mašmaššu* disappear virtually without trace.[62]

Quacks and Quacksalvers

While on the subject of medical-magical professional terminology, we noted many terms for exorcist but only one term for "doctor," *asû*. What about a word for quack or quacksalver? Akkadian appears to have none, but then again, neither does Greek.

Nevertheless, one can safely assume that quacks existed and that anyone with enough nerve could present himself as a master-apothecary. The temptation to act as a quacksalver must have been compelling, since there were no actual formal qualifications or diplomas for becoming an *asû*, except for the scions of wealthier families who studied in the scribal schools and learned to deal with medical recipes and *asûtu*. We have no way of knowing how widespread this training was among actual practitioners of medicine. Moreover, physicians were often itinerant, probably for good reason. Although locals would know if someone declared himself to be a physician without training or apprenticeship, an unscrupulous charlatan might well present himself in another city as an expert *asû*, and his foreign origins may have helped render his reputation as healer more exotic.

Furthermore, it would be difficult for an unsuspecting member of the public to know whether any prescribed medicine was legitimate or bogus. Recipes were often composed of garden herbs which were readily available and many may have relied upon a placebo effect, particularly if the patient believed that the remedy could work. Babylonian medicine, moreover, was hardly technical. Little training was required in the use of instruments, and surgery was probably performed by the barber (*gallābu*), if by anyone. The administration of drugs was no doubt most effective in the hands of someone with a convincing manner and friendly disposition, since "real" drugs sold by an *asû* and those sold by a quacksalver were probably of similar medical value.

Measures were no doubt taken by physicians to prevent poaching of patients by quacksalvers. One such measure was the common usage of *Dreckapotheke* within Babylonian medicine, which turn out to be *Decknamen* or secret names for quite ordinary drugs. The idea is that a lay person, or in this case a fraud posing as a doctor, would not be able to understand and use medical recipes, since it would become immediately obvious to the patients that the disgusting ingredients in the fake recipes, containing feces and blood, etc., did not resemble professional drug preparations. This may also be the idea behind a satire ascribed to an *aluzinnu* or "jester," in which the jester poses as an exorcist. The jester as exorcist offers obviously comic recipes of foodstuffs intended to parody hemerologies (texts identifying lucky and unlucky days of the month). A sample recipe reads as follows:

> The month of Kislimu: what is your diet? You shall dine on onager dung in bitter garlic and emmer chaff in sour milk. (Milano 2004: 252)

The satirical recipes themselves are drawn from the same *materia medica* used in medical recipes, and what emerges from the humor is that the doctor's prescriptions are thought to be as effective as ordinary household and farmyard substances.

Another Babylonian tale, intended to amuse its audience, concerned a down-and-out but resourceful fellow named Gimil-Ninurta of Nippur.[63] Having decided to exchange what little he had for one good meal, he purchased a goat, but was anxious that his relations would insist on partaking with him. He decided to offer the goat to the mayor as a gift, with the idea of being invited to dine royally with mayor. The mayor accepted the goat but threw Gimil-Ninurta out.

Gimil-Ninurta plotted his revenge against the mayor by various ruses, one of which was disguising himself as a physician from the city of Isin, the city whose patron deity was Gula, goddess of healing arts. As a visiting *asû* enjoying the reputation of the city of Isin, Gimil-Ninurta was invited to treat the mayor, who was most impressed with the physician's credentials, and even remarked that "this physician is skillful!" Gimil-Ninurta insisted on treating the mayor in a dark chamber where no one else would enter, where he tied up the mayor's hands and feet and inflicted blows on him from head to foot.

The satire of this story is based on a popular view of the physician as one who could inflict pain and suffering on a patient in the course of normal medical treatment. In other words, what the public expects from a physician's treatment is lots of pain. A good example is a typical treatment for bladder or kidney problems, which entailed the insertion of a bronze tube into the urethra, through which drugs were blown into the patient's penis, a painful procedure which probably offered little medical efficacy. Any attempt at surgery in Babylonia would also have involved the patient in a great deal of pain and discomfort, since there was little in the way of anesthesia. The Poor Man of Nippur tale shows that a quacksalver could hardly be distinguished from an *asû*, since the mayor never realizes that Gimil-Ninurta was only posing as a physician.

We usually think in terms of a bipartite division between the healing professions, a kind of therapeutic dualism: doctors versus magicians, recipe writers versus incantation experts, or *asûtu* versus *āšipūtu*. The question is whether this division between healing professionals allowed for an easy entrée for unscrupulous frauds. Another humorous composition from Babylonian scribal schools (George 1993: 63ff.) tells of a Mr Amēl-Baba, of the city of Isin, who manages to heal a patient of the effects of a dog-bite by reciting an incantation. We cannot be sure about Amēl-Baba's professional status, since he is considered to be neither

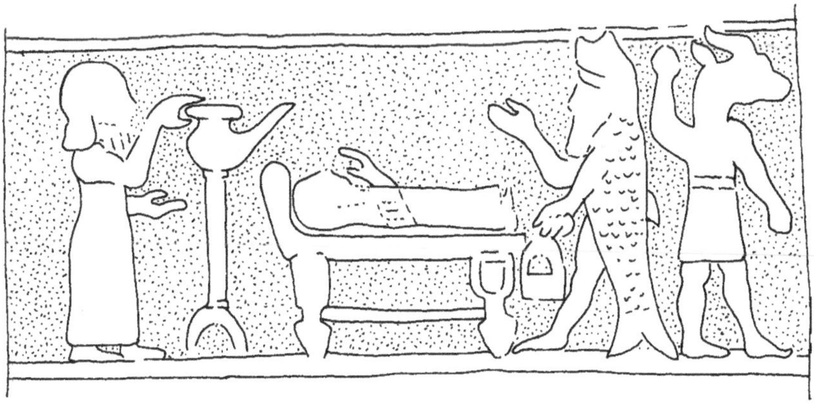

Figure 2.3 Exorcists trying to heal a patient in bed, Lamaštu-amulet (Wiggermann 2007: 107, No. 2; drawing F. A. M. Wiggermann)

physician (*asû*) nor exorcist per se, but he derives his reputation from being a priest (*šangû*) of Gula, goddess of healing. In any case, he heals his patient with an incantation, not a medical recipe. The fact that the text considers Amēl-Baba to be a quacksalver is obvious from what follows. The patient invites Amēl-Baba to his own city of Nippur, in order to pay for services rendered, but it transpires that Amēl-Baba is so ignorant that he cannot follow simple directions given to him in Sumerian, still spoken in the streets of Nippur. The image of the exorcist as scholar is exploded in this story, to the amusement of its audience, and the text itself was composed for recitation by "apprentice scribes" (*šamallû*) of Uruk.

The picture which emerges from this evidence gives a diversified view of types of Babylonian healers, with a rich vocabulary and various approaches to therapy. This should hardly surprise us, since there was no single standard qualification to distinguish objectively a "qualified" practitioner from an unscrupulous quack or inspired charismatic miracle-worker. What remains is for us to see how therapists, exorcists, and physicians appeared in actual documents and records.

3

The Politics of Medicine

Politics and medicine always go together, for several reasons. For one thing, rulers and ruling classes, like everyone else, require the services of doctors and healers, but they are in a position to afford medical services, even to the extent of inviting physicians of repute from abroad. Second, health-care provision in general is equally important to the population at large, whether provided by the state or not, and will always be a matter of public concern. The decisive question is whether the ruling powers take responsibility for public health, in the same way that charge was taken of restoring temples or maintaining public order and military activities. Finally, periodic incidences of plague or epidemic will necessarily concern the body politic as a whole.[64] The way, therefore, that society organizes (or fails to organize) health-care provisions is a matter of politics and should be seen in this light.

Medicine and healing in Mesopotamia was more or less divided between the two healing professionals, the *asû*-physician and the exorcist. Outside this system was the midwife, whose function probably went beyond childbirth to include gynecology and pediatrics, and the barber, who may have handled minor surgery. The usual assumption is that exorcists and physicians handled most aspects of healing, including diagnosis, dispensing drugs, and treating patients. Some healers at least may have charged high fees for their services, so that it would have been unlikely for ordinary members of the public to use their services (Attinger 2008: 3). Nevertheless, this type of system of health provision, provided both by the priest and the layman, was part of the fundamental structures of the state. We have no records which tell us how comprehensive or readily available such services were to ordinary citizens, although it is conceivable that the office of a priest (as exorcist) might have been part of the

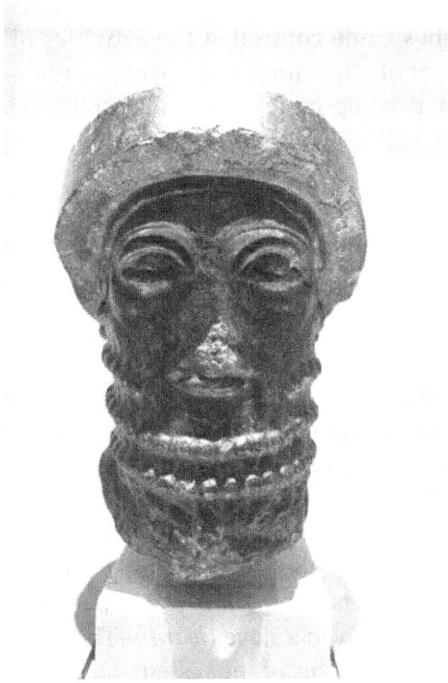

Figure 3.1 Bust of Hammurabi, king of Babylon (Musée du Louvre Sb 95; photo Florentina Badalanova Geller)

public services offered by the temple, to all classes of society. On the other hand, if the exorcist and *asû* were only affordable to upper classes of society, the poorer classes must have had other kinds of health care of which we know nothing.

Health care in Babylonia was occasionally regulated or controlled by the state, at least to an extent, and for this we turn to Hammurabi's Code, laws 206–25. We turn to the Code as a unique source of information regarding the social role of medicine during Hammurabi's reign in the early second millennium BC, following Pascal Attinger's use of this material in his excellent survey of Mesopotamian medicine.[65] We are less interested in the type of medicine per se mentioned in the Code but more interested in the status of the physician *vis-à-vis* other classes in society. In fact, the *asû*-physician is one of the few "professions" mentioned in the Code, since it was unusual in an essentially agrarian society for the affairs of a private professional entrepreneur to be regulated by law. Nothing comparable is known for the *bārû*-diviner or exorcist, whose activities were not deemed to require regulation of any sort. Hammurabi's Code controlled the activities of the *asû*-physician even to the extent of stipulating under what conditions he could charge for his services, it being understood that a physician would normally do so.

CH 206	If a man (or "gentleman," *awīlu*) has hit a man in a fight and inflicted him with a wound, that man shall take an oath, "I did not strike knowingly," and he shall be answerable (for payment) to the physician (*asû*).

The rule applied here is that someone causing personal injury to another person of equal social standing, even if he claims it to be unintentional, is responsible for the injured party's medical expenses. There is no doubt about the *asû*-physician charging for his services.

The next group of laws stipulates how much the *asû* is able to charge different social classes in society, depending upon whether the patient was a better-off "gentleman" (*awīlu*), a less well-off poor man or "commoner" (*muškēnu*), or even a slave (*wardu*). The rates of pay are variable according to the social status of the patient. On the other hand, payment for medical services ranges between 2 and 10 shekels of silver, which is the equivalent at the time of purchasing 600 to 3000 liters of barley, a considerable sum of money, which would only be affordable by upper classes in society (Attinger 2008: 3).[66]

CH 215	If a physician [*asû*] made a serious wound (incision) on a man (or "gentleman") with a bronze scalpel and healed the man, or opened a man's temple with a bronze scalpel and healed the man's eye, he shall charge 10 shekels of silver (as his fee).
CH 216	If he (the patient) is a commoner,[67] he shall charge 5 shekels of silver (as his fee).
CH 217	If he (the patient) is a gentleman's slave, the slave's owner shall give the *asû*-physician 2 shekels of silver.

This type of eye surgery described in the Code of Hammurabi was probably far from common and is never mentioned in medical texts. Rarely does a medical text, in any case, refer to the use of a scalpel. Furthermore, the risks of performing such surgery were very high, for the *asû*-physician as well as for his patient, since if anything went wrong, the physician's hand could be cut off (in theory, at least), although we never hear of such drastic punishments for medical malpractice.

CH 218	If an *asû*-physician has made a serious wound (incision) on a man with a bronze scalpel and caused the man's death, or opened a man's temple with a bronze scalpel and blinded the man's eye, they shall cut off his hand.
CH 219	If an *asû*-physician made a serious wound (incision) on a commoner's slave with a bronze scalpel and caused the slave's death, he shall replace the slave with a similar slave.
CH 220	If he opened his (the commoner's slave's) temple with a bronze scalpel and blinded his eye, he shall weigh out silver equal to half his value.

Another type of treatment regulated by Hammurabi's Code dealt with treating fractures, also an area of medicine not covered by the extant therapeutic medical corpus; there is not a single surviving treatise on how to set broken bones. A further clause governed treatment of a sore or sick tendon (*šer'ānu*), a general term for the soft tissues of the body

Figure 3.2 Seal of physician Ur-lugal-edina (Collon 1987: No. 638; drawing courtesy D. Collon)

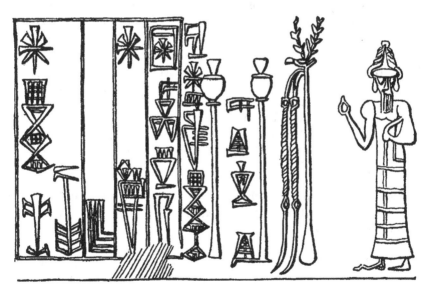

(in contrast to the bones), but in both cases the risks to doctor and patient are greatly reduced (with no threat of punishment for malpractice), and the fees are much reduced on a sliding scale. The payment for this treatment, at a rate of 5 shekels and 3 shekels respectively, is considerably cheaper than the physician's charges for surgery (CH 215–16). On the other hand, charges for healing a slave (2 shekels) are the same in both instances, and probably represented a minimum or basic fee for services rendered.

CH 221	If an *asû*-physician mended a man's broken bone or healed a sore tendon,[68] the patient shall pay the physician 5 shekels of silver.
CH 222	If he (the patient) is a commoner, he shall pay 3 shekels of silver.
CH 223	If he (the patient) is a man's slave, the slave's owner shall pay the *asû*-physician 2 shekels of silver.

There is no special term for veterinary surgeon in Akkadian and it is safe to assume that the *asû* performed this function as well. The fees are much lower, as is the penalty for malpractice. A sixth of a shekel of silver would purchase 50 liters of barley, which is a generally affordable sum as a fee (Attinger 2008: 3, 75). Note that the owner of the ox or ass is not assigned to any social class, as either *awīlu*, *muškēnu*, or *wardu*.

CH 224	If a veterinarian (lit. *asû*-physician for an ox or ass) has made a serious wound (incision) on an ox or ass and healed it, the owner of the ox shall pay the *asû*-physician one sixth (of a shekel) of silver.
CH 225	If he has made a serious wound (incision) on an ox or ass and caused its death, he shall pay one quarter of its value to the owner of the ox or ass.

The next section immediately following the laws regulating the *asû* refers to the *gallābu*-barber, who indulged in a type of surgery involving the branding of slaves.

CH 226	If a barber shaved off the mark of a slave without an owner (and) not his own, they shall cut off that barber's hand.

Although no fee is stipulated, the barber faces the same malpractice penalty as the *asû*, in having his hand cut off. The barber may have served as a cheaper surgeon than the *asû*, used specifically for matters dealing with slaves, but later dropped out of the medical record.[69] This may be because of the lack of any real records dealing with surgery, which was probably not considered to belong to the art of medicine, as in medieval Europe. Nevertheless, it is conceivable that the barber continued to offer some type of medical services to lower classes in society in later periods.

The Code of Hammurabi ends in an epilogue containing a medical curse against anyone who defaces it:

CH E 50ff.	May Ninkarak (Gula) daughter of Anu, who speaks in my favor in the Ekur temple, make a serious illness break out in his limbs, a malicious demon[70] or a grievous wound (*simmu*) which cannot be soothed, which no *asû*-physician knows anything about nor can treat with bandages, and like the bite of death cannot be eradicated.

The *asû*-physician is faced here with disease and lesions, which he cannot diagnose, recognize, or treat, all caused by the goddess Gula, who is normally the patron goddess of healing. Like the exorcist, the physician was also dependant upon gods for his ability to treat patients, and gods could equally prevent such healing if the patient was morally culpable. The ultimate basis for healing and illness was ascribed to divine will, a notion shared by both physician and exorcist.

What is clear, however, is that the *exorcist* as healer is never mentioned in Hammurabi's Code, and it is difficult to know why this is so. One reason might be that the social status of the *asû*-physician was higher in this period than that of his exorcist colleague, although as a priest one might imagine that an exorcist commanded respect. The fact that the exorcist was associated with the temple may also have been a factor in his exclusion from the Code, which deals primarily with civil law associated with the palace rather than cultic regulations associated with the temple. One final suggestion as to why the physician is exclusively mentioned in the Code is because of the type of medicine specified, related to surgery, setting bones, and veterinary medicine, rather than the pharmacological remedies which we find in our medical corpus, for which legal regulation was not deemed to be necessary. In addition to controlling how much the physician could charge, it is clear that the Code seeks to protect the public from the unlucky or unscrupulous doctor who harms his patient, which was obviously seen as a potential threat to society.

Letters from the Kingdom of Mari (Syria), Eighteenth Century BC

One of the elusive aspects of ancient medicine is the encounter between doctor and patient, which was a special relationship, even if the encounter may not have been held strictly in private but was witnessed by other members of the family. This dialogue between doctor and patient usually concerned the general welfare, habits, pains, bodily functions, and state of mind of the patient. Although ancient medical literature is replete with instructions to the physician and with general reports of what physicians have found when meeting patients, rarely do we get actual records of an actual interview between doctor and patient.

One of the unique characteristics of Akkadian administrative archives is the large quantity of official and private letters which survive, thanks to the durable nature of the clay upon which they were written, and a substantial number of these letters refer to meetings between a doctor and his patient. The earliest of such archives containing medical information is to be found in the city of Mari, in Syria, during the eighteenth century BC, representing chancery documents from the royal palace of Mari. Mari was a major capital of a kingdom which dominated northern Syria in the third millennium and well into the second millennium BC. By lucky chance, a number of letters refer to physicians (the *asû*), probably in the employ of the royal palace, who were asked to treat patients in the royal circle.[71]

The most prominent medical practitioner appearing in the Mari archives was the *asû*-doctor and sometimes surgeon.[72] Although Mari chancery letters refer to a cadre of palace doctors as part of the state bureaucracy,[73] nonetheless the physicians most highly prized and recommended were brought from a neighboring country, which is a frequently recurring pattern among palace physicians.

One letter sent between members of the ruling family refers to a particular physician and the drugs he prescribed:

> Say to Yasmah-Addu, thus speaks Išme-Dagan, your brother:
>
> The drugs,[74] from which your physician (*asû*) made me a plaster, are excellent. Whenever a sore (*simmu*)[75] occurs, this plant (accompanying the letter) will heal it immediately.
>
> Here now I have sent you Samsi-Addu-tukultī, an apprentice *asû*, so that he promptly notes (the effects of) this plant. Send him back to me. (Durand 2002: 305 No. 65 = ARM 4 65)

The ailment concerned is a skin disease of some type, for which a successful remedy was found using the external application of plants, although how many and which plants are not specified. The disease itself, *simmu*, can refer to sores, wounds, or many types of skin ailments, which were to be treated by external applications or bandages. The relief from *simmu* afforded by the plaster is immediate. It was a chief physician (whose name is not recorded) who prepared the medication, while the apprentice or junior physician was charged with the application of the remedy.[76] We have no way of knowing what happens if the remedy does not produce the desired effect, but in any case the apprentice-physician was not to be blamed.

A second important letter sent to the King of Mari concerns fever.

> Speak to my Lord, thus (speaks) Dariš-libur, your servant.
>
> Regarding the plants (employed) against "sun-fever," of the physician (*asû*) from Mardamân and of the staff physician, about which the Lord has written to me. I have sent their plants, which were gathered on a mountain, under seal with my signature to my Lord, and (I have sent) these physicians with La-gamal-abum, together with their plants.
>
> My Lord has already tried the remedy for "sun-fever" of the staff physician, but I have (also) tried the remedy for "sun-fever" of the Mardamân physician and it is good. I tried it many times together with Hammi-šagiš and it is good. Abu-ma-nasi (also) drank it and it was good.
>
> Now for the moment, it isn't necessary that we have my Lord drink a mixture of these drugs. Let him take these drugs separately, and let someone in charge administer the potion to my Lord. (Durand 2002: 306 = Finet 1957: 134f.)

This letter contrasts the recommendations of the local "staff-physician" with the more exotic and perhaps more respected foreign physician from a distant place, Mardamân. The medical problem in question is *himiṭ ṣēti*, a fever which may also be related to sunlight or sunstroke.[77] The medical novelty in this letter is the opposition between drinking a cocktail of "mixed" drugs in contrast to "simples," that is each drug or plant being taken individually to see if it is effective or not. This is an early indication within Babylonian medicine of rudimentary "trial and error" and represents a rational approach to drug therapy. This is not to say that the Babylonian *asû* had anything resembling a laboratory in his house where he could test the efficacy of drugs, or even that a Babylonian physician systematically recorded the effect of any drug on a patient; no extant medical texts describe the actual testing of a drug, either on humans or on animals. We do get a frequent remark in later tablets attesting that a recipe has been "tested" (*bulṭu latku*), but the practicalities behind this expression are never explained. How any drug was "tested," or by whom, or under what conditions, is never recorded.

This letter alludes to the matter of confidence in the physician, which may have had important psychological benefits for healing the patient. The presence of a foreign physician, whose services were no doubt more expensive, appears to be more attractive than the services of the "staff physician," who was part of the existing court bureaucracy. The very existence of a court staff physician is noteworthy, but importing a foreign physician is known from many other examples, usually at a royal court. The example from our Mari letter is an early example of this phenomenon.

A foreign physician appears in another Mari letter:

> A youth who is in my service is ill, and a sore has appeared below his ear which has produced an abscess. The two *asû*-physicians who are at my disposal have bandaged it but his *simmu* (sore) hasn't changed. Now, it is imperative that my Lord send me a Mardamân-physician or else a medical expert so that he examines the youth's lesion (*simmu*) and bandages it so that his lesion will not persist. (Finet 1957: 131 = Durand 1988: 552)

Local physicians are again compared unfavorably with physicians brought from afar or an "expert" (*asû hakammu*), whose expertise is considered superior to that of local doctors. The writer of the letter is certain, moreover, that better medical advice will cure the lad. The condition to be treated is also a *simmu*, described here as a sore on the ear which has produced an abscess (lit. issue), probably containing pus.[78] The recommended local treatment was a bandage, not radically different from that recommended by the foreign or expert physicians.

Another disease attested at Mari was *bennu*, "seizure," a broad term including epilepsy. One court letter refers to a woman, Šimatum, described as having been "seized" by an angry god, who had mutilated her fingers and had caused her to suffer from *bennu* (Durand 1988: 553 No. 312). Since there is no reference in the letter to her seeing a doctor, we can assume that the reference to "seizure" is layman's terminology rather than a professional medical diagnosis.

Mari letters refer to *ziqtu*, a medical condition affecting the foot, which is a disease known from later medical texts (Durand 1988: 553, 567). The relevant part of one letter reads,

> When the [letter] of my Lord was received, on that day I was ready to depart, but *ziqtum* (severe pain) arose in my foot, (while) in the palace,[79]

> in all of my sinews, right into the sole of my foot below and throbbing upwards right into my belly. ... In five days, my foot will be healed. (Durand 1988: No. 266)

The writer of this letter describes his own illness, similar to how a patient would discuss his condition with his doctor; technically, the patient's own observations are "signs," while those of the doctor are "symptoms." The word used to describe the condition, *ziqtu*, literally means a "bite,"[80] and in this case the author could have used the word metaphorically, meaning a "stinging sensation" appeared in his foot, although in later medical texts the technical term refers specifically to a painful condition affecting the skin. The correspondent, writing to the king Yasmah-Addu, expects to be healed within five days, although we have no way of knowing upon what his prognosis is based. Without other corroborative evidence, it is best to assume that there is no technical medical terminology or professional judgment expressed in this letter.

One letter addressed to the Mari king (probably Zimri-Lim) cites a report by an administrator who complained directly to Hammurabi that "oil is not being applied to patients" and "their faces are not being examined" (Durand 1988: No. 273). Both procedures refer to standard medical practice. Various oils served as a common soothing agent for all kinds of sores and ailments, and examining the face of a patient was a basic tenet of prognosis and diagnosis, exemplified in prognostic omens in the Diagnostic Handbook. What is interesting in this letter is not the medical information, but rather the fact that basic medical provisions, including *materia medica*, were expected to be provided by the king or society in general. A report sent back to Hammurabi in Babylon about poor health-care in the region was a potential source of embarrassment and a bad reflection on the King of Mari.

There was a limit, however, to what the king could provide. One letter from Mari refers to the case of a doctor (*asû*) who refused to come to Mari to work for Yasmah-Addu, the king (Durand 1988: No. 267). The doctor's brother wrote to explain that the doctor had previously lived at Mari for three years and lived in poverty, and the writer wanted to know what his doctor brother would be given by way of support. Even assuming that the claims made in this letter are somewhat exaggerated, what surprises us is the independence of a physician who felt able to refuse the king's invitation of service. Under these circumstances, it seems that doctors were influential enough to resist being regulated or controlled by royal authority.[81]

Physicians in Babylonia (Eighteenth–Seventeenth Century BC)

Evidence for exorcists in this period is sparse, and what few references we have to healing professionals usually mention the *asû*-physician only. Two contracts from the city of Larsa, for instance, provide information from daily life about the local *asû*-physician, who was involved in the sale of a house. One contract, dating from the fifteenth day of the sixth month of the sixth year of king Samsuiluna (c. 1743 BC), documents the sale of a house which borders on a temple of Šamaš; the house is being sold by an *asû*, Apil-ilišu, and a second contract dating from exactly one month later documents the sale of a neighboring property (Farber 1999: 135–40). The exceptional feature of these documents is that eight witnesses to one contract are high-ranking priests or temple administrators from the Šamaš Temple,[82] although the vendor, an *asû*, is a layman.[83] It is clear from these two documents that the vendor, the physician Apil-ilišu, was a successful and respected professional within his local community.

Second-Millennium BC Medical Corpus

Since archival records of the second millennium give prominence to the physician over the exorcist in most health matters, it would be instructive to look for confirmation in an actual medical text from the so-called Old Babylonian period. We must bear in mind that first-millennium medical texts usually contain a mixture of therapeutic recipes and incantations, showing the considerable influence of magic on medicine in later periods.

The following medical tablet from Nippur, dating roughly from the eighteenth century BC, includes recipes for a variety of ailments, and provides a very different picture of medicine from what we find in later medical literature.

1 If a man is behexed, you dry out *armanum*, red salt,
2 kidney of a sheep which has not yet tasted grass,
3 (and) *ernīnum*-plant, he will eat (them) and get better.[84]

---

4 If a man suffers from jaundice,
5 you soak licorice root in milk,
6 you leave it out overnight (lit. under the stars), you blend it
7 in pressed oil, have him drink it and he will get better.

---

8 If a man (has) a worm in his tooth,
9 you crush "sailor's excrement"[85] in pressed oil;
10 if it is a tooth on the right which aches,
11 you pour (the oil) on a tooth on the left and he will get better.
12 If it is tooth on the left which aches,
13 you pour (the oil) on a tooth on the right and he will get better.

---

14 If a man is covered with red spots, you blend malt-flour
15 in pressed oil in equal measures,
16 you apply (it on the patient) and he will get better.
17 If he does not recover, you apply a hot *tincture* and he will get better.
18 If he does not recover, you apply hot *tuhhu*-residue and he will get better.

---

19 If a man has been stung by a scorpion,
20 you apply bull's saliva and he will get better.

---

21 If a man's eyes are unwell, you strain (through a cloth) *hartitu*(-red flower),
22 you apply it (as a bandage) and he will get better.

---

23 If a man is burning up with "sun-fever," you blend *tillaqurdu*,
24 cinders, groats-flour, *maštakal*,
25 and old brick in refined oil,
26 and [..... and he will get better].

---

27 If a man is ... [.........................
28 [...

Reverse

29 If a man is behexed? [...........................]
30 you apply (the fruit) of *libāru* against fever [and he will get better].

---

31 If a man's forehead is *thick*,
32 you apply tamarisk-seed and [he will get better].

---

33 If a man is bitten by a dog, it being the case that a "puppy" is not born,[86]
34 you apply *maštakal* and *šakirūtu* in ghee,
35 he will consume it and get better.

---

37 If a man (has) a worm in his tooth,
38 you dry out the peel of [....], apply it and he will get better.

---

39 If a man's innards are inflamed,
40 he drinks black cumin in best-quality oil and he will get better.

41 If a man is behexed, he drinks *nuhurtu* root (dissolved)
42 in refined oil and he will get better.

43 If a man is ill in the anus, you dry out raw meat and (roast it),
44 you blend it with refined oil, you cool it down and he will get better.
45 If afterwards an abscess stings him, you soak the plucked wool
46 in boiled tincture, (apply it) and he will get better.

47 If a man's feet "lick the ground,"
48 you heat up water in a cauldron and bathe him,
49 after he vomits, you cool (him) down with oil and he will get better.

50 If a man head is burning up with "sun-fever,"
51 you press his head with powder,
52 you pour oil (on him) and he will get better.
53 If he is hot (feverish), you add oil and he will get better.

54 If a man is constantly inflamed in his internal organs,
55 he drinks *nīnû* in beer and he will get better. (*BAM* 393)

The first thing to notice is that this recipe contains no magic and not a single incantation. The tablet is not arranged in a head-to-foot format, which we expect from first-millennium BC diagnostic texts, but it associates diseases according to other organizing principles. The text alternates between diseases for which a cause has been determined (such as witchcraft, worm in a tooth, a dog-bite, etc.) and other diseases for which no cause is known (sick eyes, swollen chest); in the latter case, it is difficult to differentiate between a disease and its symptoms (Geller 2006: 10; Schwemer 2007: 28 n. 24).

If we compare this medical text, from the early second millennium, with medical matters raised in royal correspondence, we find that technical disease terminology of the medical corpus is not reflected in the layman's language of contemporary letters, but the lack of incantations within recipes supports the assumed primary medical role in this period of the *asû* over the exorcist.

Epidemics

There were times when the offices of the exorcist may have been in demand, especially during epidemics, which are occasionally mentioned in Mari letters (Durand 1988: 544–9). According to one letter sent to the king, Yasmah-Addu, an epidemic affecting the neighboring city of Tuttul caused many people to be ill, but with few deaths, while in another city, Dunnum, at least 20 persons were reported to have died from the pest, with the result that many people abandoned the city for the mountains. Mari, on the other hand, is reported to have been spared from this outbreak (Durand 1988: 561 No. 259). Similarly, a second letter to Yasmah-Addu reports an outbreak of disease in the cities of Zurubbân and Zapad, two cities not in immediate proximity to each other, indicating on this occasion a more widespread epidemic (Durand 1988: 563 No. 261). Another letter addressed to Yasmah-Addu reports that the epidemic, (called here "the hand of the god," a term we also encounter in medical texts), had resulted in the deaths of weavers, craftsmen, and agricultural workers (Durand 1988: 565 No. 264). It is possible that these workers, as part of the corvée, lived and worked in close quarters and in poor conditions, which encouraged the spread of disease.

It is not clear what measures could be taken to combat an epidemic, other than abandoning the site. One letter to Yasmah-Addu explains that the epidemic had passed but survivors had delayed in burying the dead until the proper omens had been taken (Durand 1988: 564 No. 263), indicating that diviners were also present, in addition to exorcists and lamentation priests. Speedy burial of the dead and ritual purification were probably the only defense against contagious diseases, and the acts of purification (through washing and burning) known from ritual texts may have reduced the chance of further infection, if the disease was caused by bacteria. After the burials had taken place, the exorcists and lamentation priests purified the city (Durand 1988: 564), but the activities of the *asû* are not mentioned in this connection in the Mari archives, perhaps because the *asû* would have little to offer by way of effective remedies.

Generally, however, within the extensive corpus of Mari letters and letters from Babylonia proper, as well as contracts and law codes, we find few references to exorcists, and matters dealing with medicine appear to be in the hands of the *asû*-physician. This is not coincidental, since archives from Mari and elsewhere are palace rather than temple archives, in which case we should not be surprised to find the secular *asû*-physician, who was not a priest, rather than the reported activities of the temple-associated exorcist. Moreover, we have little information about exorcists, since most early-second-millennium temple records refer more commonly to the *pašīšu* or išib/*išippu*, two types of purification priests,[87] titles which later mostly fall out of use. This represents a troubling disjuncture in our documentation, since we have a wealth of incantations from the second millennium BC (see Cunningham 1997: 131–59), but only a very few medical texts, and even fewer medical texts from the third millennium (Attinger 2008: 9–18). On the other hand, what data we have seems to indicate that the *asû* was the key medical figure of this period, in Mesopotamia itself, as well as in Syria.

Middle Babylonian Letters (c. Fifteenth Century BC)

Another group of letters from several hundred years later in the latter half of the second millennium BC offers a further opportunity to eavesdrop on the therapist–patient relationship, although this time in Babylonia itself, rather than in Mari. The letters come from the city of Nippur, in the heart of Babylonia, and were composed by several different writers, although the majority of letters appear to have been written by one Šumu-libši, who never describes himself as an *asû*, nor do his colleagues. One assumes that they are physicians because their letters describe ill patients and treatments recommended for their recovery. The question of Šumu-libši's professional status is not straightforward, since this particular group of tablets belongs to temple archives, from where we might expect to find records of the exorcist rather than *asû*. Šumu-libši was either an exorcist with serious medical expertise or an *asû*-physician who was called in to treat temple personnel.

One of Šumu-libši's letters describes a female patient, known only as "Ayyāru's daughter," who suffered from an undescribed illness, but for which the treatment was a poultice to be applied at night (Parpola 1983: 492). On this occasion, however, the writer reports that the girl had felt better and had fallen asleep, without anyone applying her nightly poultice. She asked for the bandage in the morning because she was not feeling well, with the implication being that the relapse was caused by the lack of proper treatment. Šumu-libši promised to investigate. One key phrase in this letter refers to the girl's state of health, "whereas before she was feeling much better, now she does not feel well."[88]

In a second letter, Šumu-libši describes the symptoms of "Muštālu's daughter" (Parpola 1983: 493). Šumu-libši reports that the girl suffered from an attack of fever (*ummu*) in the night, but at first light he had given her an unspecified "drug" (*šammu*). The result was that the fever was "constant" (*mithar*), that is, not vacillating between high and low temperatures. Šumu-libši also reports that her feet are cool, and that while she had previously been coughing, she no longer does so.[89]

It appears that both of these girls were suffering from the same ailment, as is shown by a third letter from Šumu-libši, according to which the "inflammations" on the chest of both girls have given off "perspiration" (Parpola 1983: 493). It then turns out that the same is happening with other girls, such as the daughters of messieurs Kuri, Ilī-ippašra, and Ahuni, but the daughters of two ladies, Babati and Bitti, are in a better state; their "inflammations" produce no "perspiration." He reports that these latter two are in stable health.

A subsequent letter from Šumu-libši from the same archive follows on from the first two in sequence (Parpola 1983: 494), since he reports that inflammations of Muštālu's daughter are healed and she no longer coughs, although he makes no reference to Ayyāru's daughter. He reports on the other patients as well, all female: the daughters of Kuri and Ahuni are healed[90] and can return to their training,[91] although a new patient, Eṭirtu, now shows symptoms of the same disease. Furthermore, Ilī-ippašra's daughter has an inflammation showing a reddish discoloration, although her disease appears to have improved.[92] Babati's daughter, mentioned as improving in a previous letter, is now not doing well, since she continues to cough and suffer from inflammation.

The combination of symptoms gives a rough idea of the nature of the illness which had spread among a group of female musicians living or working in the same quarters. The condition is characterized by the presence of "inflammations" occurring on the chest or ribs or back. Other symptoms are coughing and fever. A final letter of Šumu-libši reports his observations over a two-day period in which he notes that his patient (probably a woman, Eṭirtu) was seized by fever (*ummu*), and she was unable to finish eating a single meal with porridge (*papassu*), a type of barley gruel which was medicinal (Parpola 1983: 495). These symptoms probably reflect an infectious disease.

Šumu-libši also refers to the services of his colleague, one Bēlum-balāṭi,[93] who treated Huttirmu's daughter. In fact, we have a remarkable letter from Bēlum-balāṭi, reporting on his treatment. A patient suffering from a chest condition required a poultice and a potion for the windpipes. For a second patient, Bēlum-balāṭi justified his diagnosis by quoting the incipit of a medical text: *šum-ma* LÚ *ki-ma ek-ke-*⸢*tú*⸣ [*ik-kal-šú*], "if a man (suffers) when a skin disease [causes him pain]." Bēlum-balāṭi's letter goes on to complain that he cannot properly prescribe a bandage because one essential ingredient was unavailable:

> When I prescribed a bandage for him, the *ašû*-plant was missing, and my Lord knows that if (even) one herb is missing, he will not get better. (Parpola 1983: 495 12–15)

The exactitude of this remark is impressive, with its assertion that a compound medical recipe made up of several drugs is ineffective unless all active ingredients are present. On the other hand, the missing drug, *ašû*, was rather commonplace and used in a variety of different recipes, and does not appear to be either exotic or rare. The fact that Bēlum-balāṭi quotes a medical incipit and cites a rule about recipes – that no ingredient can be omitted – is no doubt intended to prove his medical qualifications.[94]

This same writer, Bēlum-balāṭi, discusses a further case of a woman suffering from a cough, for which the treatment caused unwanted side-effects, and she now suffers from some kind of abdominal cramps (*kīs libbi*), for which yet another potion had to be prescribed. This letter is an important witness to how drug preparations developed from "simples" (one drug to treat one disease) into compound recipes, some later containing as many as 90 different drugs. Acting as an apothecary, the ancient physician probably prescribed a drug and noticed whether it produced any undesired side-effects, and, if so, then the recipe had to be altered to treat the side-effects as well.[95] Another incentive to create compound recipes came from patients, who may have thought compound recipes more effective than a single-ingredient drug.[96] This may be the reason why Bēlum-balāṭi's letter ends with a request list of 12 urgently required drugs, many of which can be identified in the later medical corpus.[97]

Letters and documents from Nippur and Boghazkoy provide unparalleled data about the practice of medicine in the second millennium BC, and they predominantly refer to the activities of the *asû* rather than the exorcist. Although the orientation of the archives (palace versus temple) might explain the more frequent references to physician over exorcist, another explanation is possible. The role of exorcist and physician throughout the second millennium most likely reflected a clear division of responsibility and tasks, with the exorcist essentially magico-religious in his orientation and the physician's interests being magico-medical. This clear division, however, did not persist through the next millennium, when we see how roles of exorcist and physician radically change during the course of time.

Literary Hypochondria

In addition to a large corpus of Assyrian and Babylonian letters dealing with medical matters, we have reports of patients complaining about their illnesses or mental distress. One is in the form of a famous literary autobiographical composition known as *Ludlul bēl nēmeqi*, the Poem of the Righteous Sufferer, ascribed to the Babylonian courtier Šubši-mešrê-Šakkan, who would have flourished in the late second millennium BC (Lambert 1967: 21–62; Foster 2007: 32–4). The writer complains that he suffers from slander and treachery, but that none of the professionals (diviners, dream interpreters, or *mašmaššu*-exorcists) offered helpful advice; the author is referring to various kinds of rituals and treatments designed to deal with such problems. He then lists the various illnesses from which he suffers, including headache, cough, chills, infection, fevers, and paralysis, among others, for which neither the diviner nor the exorcist provides a satisfactory diagnosis. Finally, however, an exorcist sent by Marduk manages to effect a cure. The literary nature of this poem, which remained popular throughout the first millennium BC, makes it unlikely to have been based upon any identifiable actual person or situation. On the other hand, if the poem is based on real life, only a king or senior court official would have been able to afford to commission a text of such literary value.

A second text comes from a recently excavated stele from Syria, from one of the banks of the Upper Euphrates, in the vicinity of Terqa and Dura-Europus, dating from approximately the eighth century BC. In this stele, the local ruler, Adad-bēl-ardi, describes his miseries and illnesses in remarkable detail, in language reminiscent of the Poem of the Righteous Sufferer.[98] He begins by recounting his early childhood illness, which included sores covering his whole body. Among other ailments of the head and neck, he developed blurred vision and arthritis-like symptoms in his hands.

> Day and night, sleep afforded my feet no rest,
> I stopped (normal) human nourishment, I became like a dead man.

He explains that despite making offerings to gods, he received no succor or favorable attention, even from his own personal god. He finally recounts that,

> I had no relief from dreams or divination. I did not reach to using medicine,
> (nor) to the exorcist casting spells, and my head was pushed away.

This unusual stele is a unique "case history" from Mesopotamia, recording the patient's own report of his medical condition and referring to himself by name. The stele is a personal prayer addressed to Nabû, and in many ways resembles the woes expressed by Šubši-mešrê-Šakkan. The specific illnesses of which the writer complains are not the

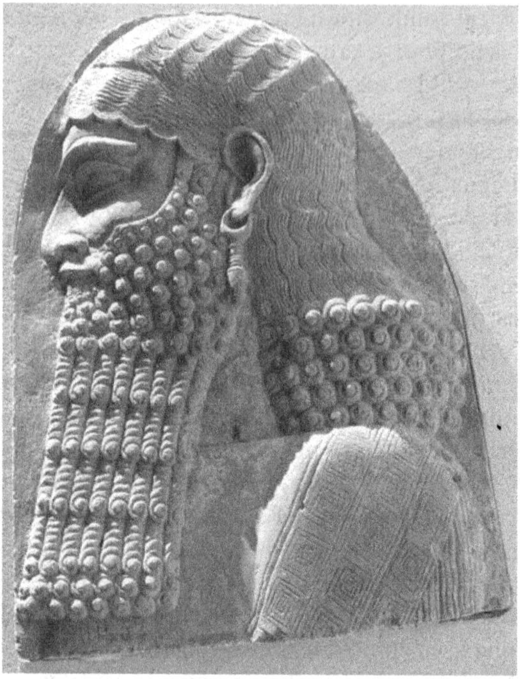

Figure 3.3 Bust of an Assyrian courtier (Musée du Louvre; photo Florentina Badalanova Geller)

technical disease terms found in the extensive Babylonian medical corpus. The first of these, *ṣibit nakkapti*, refers to an attack of the temples, perhaps referring to migraine. The second condition is labeled *sihlu*, which means "piercing pain," although the term is not used for acute pain in the medical corpus. This text is a description, in layman's words, of chronic illness which has afflicted the patient since childhood. The stele ends with a plea to the gods to alleviate his illness, and the complaints about ineffective remedies probably show the limited range of therapies available in the seventh century BC, even to a member of the ruling class.[99]

Such autobiographical accounts of personal illness are rare but not entirely unique in the classical world. One celebrated example is the second century AD account of Aelius Aristides, who at one time was a patient of Galen (Nutton 2004: 277–9; Lloyd 2003: 213–15). A notorious hypochondriac, Aristides kept a full record of his many illnesses. According to his *Sacred Tales*, Aristides was critical of his many doctors and turned to Asclepius for help, much as Adad-bēl-ardi turned to the gods after rejecting the services of doctors and exorcists.

Neo-Assyrian Court Letters

We have many letters from Assyrian and Babylonian *savants* at the Assyrian court corresponding with the kings Esarhaddon and Assurbanipal, during the years of their respective reigns (681–c. 630 BC). These letters provide invaluable information about how medicine and healing magic was practiced in everyday life, at least at the royal court. There can also be little doubt about the political importance of these letters, since physicians and exorcists, as well as diviners, lamentation priests, and scribes, all enjoyed royal patronage and were supported by the king. It is also abundantly clear that decisions affecting the king, including matters dealing with his private health, were also affairs of state affecting the country as a whole.

Scholars at the Assyrian court needed to justify their appointments. The letters mention exorcist (*mašmaššu*), physician (*asû*), lamentation singer (*kalû*), scribe (*ṭupšarru*), and diviner (*bārû*). Two of these, the exorcist and lamentation singer, also functioned as priests, although whether in a dual capacity – as priests working in the palace – is difficult to say. The idea of priests on secondment to the palace would not necessarily be a conflict of interests, but the converse was also possible, i.e. laymen working in the temple.[100] In effect, the exorcist and lamentation priests, in the late first millennium BC, could have had a broader range of professional options than either the *asû*-physician or *bārû*-diviner, as non-priests.

One important letter among the court correspondence (SAA 10 160) was written by Marduk-šāpik-zēri, probably to Assurbanipal (see Hunger 1987: 162).[101] The king claimed himself to be generally better versed in scribal arts than any of his predecessors (Hunger 1968: No. 329), including specialized disciplines such as extispicy (*bārûtu*) (Hunger 1968: No. 325), and even if this is an exaggeration, scribes within his court would have to take these claims into consideration. If Assurbanipal valued his own expertise in technical matters so highly, scribes would no doubt have to claim superior abilities in order to be appointed to work in the royal administration. This is what we find in a letter of Marduk-šāpik-zēri in which he applies for a position within the palace administration for himself and for his hand-picked team of 20 scholars (SAA 10 160). The writer is otherwise unknown in administrative archives, which could mean that his application failed. In any case, he begins his letter by showing off his abilities in interpreting celestial omens, probably based upon the well-known series, Enūma-Anu-Enlil (for which, see Rochberg 2004: 66–78). To display his skill, Marduk-šāpik-zēri reinterprets a potentially bad omen about silting up of the Tigris and Euphrates and declares the omen to be favorable, since the logogram (IDIM) for "silt" (*sakīku*) can also mean "well" or "spring" (*nagbu*), hence portending prosperity rather than catastrophe. Marduk-šāpik-zēri then goes on to give his credentials, being the son of a *kalû*-priest, but also having learned various purification rituals and even diagnosis (examining "healthy and sick flesh"), which implies that he had mastered healing arts in addition to physiognomic and standard omens. There is no doubt about the comprehensive nature of Marduk-šāpik-zēri's education, if what he writes is correct.

There are some troubling aspects to this letter. Among his team of experts whom Marduk-šāpik-zēri recommends to the king's services, several individuals are referred to as "refugee[s] (*halqu*) from Assyria," which might make sense if these scholars had escaped from Assyria to Babylonia during the revolt of Šamaš-šuma-ukin against Assurbanipal in 652 BC.[102] The fact that Marduk-šāpik-zēri could have been on the losing side in the revolt (i.e Babylonia) may explain why neither he nor his comrades are heard of again.

The other question is whether this letter makes a realistic or exaggerated case for the competence of Marduk-šāpik-zēri and his cronies. One of the scholars named Aqrea, a refugee from Assyria, had been a slave, since his face and hand had been branded with his owner's name; nevertheless he was described as someone accomplished in the art of exorcism (*āšipūtu*) (SAA 10 160: 11). Unlike Greek slaves in Rome, there is no tradition in Mesopotamia of slaves being scholars.[103] Most of the other members of the group were trained in a single discipline, either lamentations (*kalûtu*) or exorcism (*āšipūtu*), although some scholars were claimed to have mastered more than one area of study. One exception is another refugee from Assyria, a certain Kudurru, who had studied scribal arts (*ṭupšarrūtu*) and exorcism (*āšipūtu*), in addition to being competent in one other discipline (possibly divination). Another scholar with the same name, Kudurru, could handle both terrestrial and celestial omens, a plausible combination. On the other hand, normally scribes who dealt with celestial omens were priests,[104] while terrestrial omens were handled by non-priests (*bārû*). Finally, one scholar (whose name is lost) among this group had emigrated from Elam, probably as a result of wars between Assurbanipal and Elam at this time. He had mastered extispicy and celestial omens, as well as Sumerian esoteric literature and commentary texts, and he could be classed as a genuine academic (SAA 10 160 reverse 1–3).

The only claims which appear to be extraordinary are those made by Marduk-šāpik-zēri about his own competence, since the list of his accomplishments reads like a catalogue of the entire school curriculum. He never actually refers to his own professional status, either as a *kalû* or *mašmaššu* or *ṭupšarru*. It may be that even if one had studied these disciplines, one was not entitled to refer to oneself as a *kalû* or *mašmaššu* or *ṭupšarru* until one held an actual appointment in either a temple or palace bureaucracy, since there were no diplomas or recognized academic or professional qualifications.[105] One could only establish credentials as a professional by acting in a professional capacity. But what happened with those professions, such as *asû* or *barû*, which had no priestly status to support professional qualifications? We can only assume that one's reputation was based upon successful results. This may be why Marduk-šāpik-zēri's letter began with his own interpretation of celestial omens, by which he hoped to convince the king of his professional competence.

Once appointed to the royal court, questions of power and status within the state bureaucracy would naturally surface. One of the problems facing courtiers was the corvée or *ilku*-service, which affected scholars as well as other members of society. Two letters, one from an *asû* (in fact, the King's Physician) and another from a scribe, complain about the corvée obligation imposed upon them, despite their responsibilities at court (SAA 10 324 and 143). Professionals at court objected to the fact that they were still subject to normal tax obligations.

Since temple personnel had *ilku*-obligations to the temple,[106] we find exorcists also complaining about their working conditions and scale of remuneration. It was not unusual, in fact, for exorcists to complain to the king. One such complaint dates from a letter written by the Chief Exorcist, Adad-šumu-uṣur. He wrote to Esarhaddon twice in 667 BC (SAA 10 224) to ask that his son Urad-Gula be reinstated at court, and his petitions seemed to have worked, since letters dating from a year later thank the king for allowing Adad-šumu-uṣur's entire family to act as royal exorcists (SAA 10 227).[107] Such unabashed nepotism is not surprising, since it is likely that Adad-šumu-uṣur was part of a large family of priests, all of whom shared the occupation of exorcist (Jean 2006: 190). Urad-Gula succeeded his father as Chief Exorcist,[108] but he, too, wrote to the king with complaints. Perhaps he, like his father, was subject to depression, and like his father did not

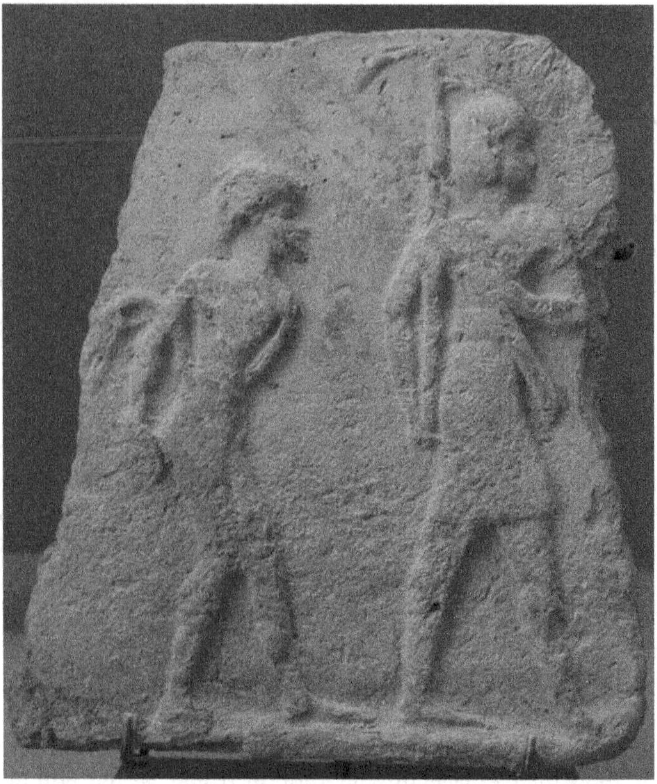

Figure 3.4 Ceramic plaque showing healer and patient, second millennium BC (Musée du Louvre AO 6622; photo Florentina Badalanova Geller)

hesitate to inform the king of his state of mind, but in any case the tone of the letter shows how influential and virtually unassailable was the position of a high-ranking exorcist at court (Glassner 2007: 136–8).

Urad-Gula's lengthy letter to Assurbanipal (SAA 10 294) is a catalogue of his lifetime woes, beginning with his impoverished early years, and ending with his impoverished present state. The tone of familiarity in Urad-Gula's letter to Assurbanipal is impressive. In his second letter (SAA 10 289), Urad-Gula complains about a rival receiving financial benefits, while he received nothing. Compared to other letters of complaint (e.g. SAA 10 171 and 173), those of Urad-Gula display a sense of security which may be a general reflection on the status of the *mašmaššu* within the Assyrian court, having unparalleled influence over the king. One attractive suggestion is that Urad-Gula had been one of Assurbanipal's personal tutors (Jean 2006: 118).. The relationship between the chief *mašmaššu* and the king may have been one of patronage, through which Urad-Gula's father requested a position for his son, and through which Urad-Gula complained to the king from a sense of entitlement (Westbrook 2005: 222f.). In any case, the position of Chief Exorcist seems to been more secure than that of other scholars.[109] By contrast the letters of the Chief Physician (*asû*) are businesslike and formal, showing no sense of familiarity or personal relations with the king, and in fact we only have one archive of a royal physician among the many court letters.

Urad-Nanaya, Chief Physician to Esarhaddon

Esarhaddon's Chief Physician, Urad-Nanaya, was not in a particularly advantageous position at the Assyrian royal court, since he faced formidable rivals and competition. His most immediate rival was the Chief Exorcist, Adad-šumu-uṣur, who had a much closer personal relationship with the king, and it was often the case that the Chief Exorcist offered medical advice which was similar to that which he himself gave. Urad-Nanaya took the opportunity on one occasion of complaining about Adad-šumu-uṣur, who had prohibited the princes, Assurbanipal and Šamaš-šuma-ukin, from going outside before the twenty-second of Tishri (SAA 10 314 and 328).[110] In any case, Urad-Nanaya challenged this prohibition, insisting that Adad-šumu-uṣur be questioned regarding an unfavorable omen behind his ruling, with Adad-šumu-uṣur being forced to admit that there was none. It is easy to envisage disagreements between the two professions regarding interpretations of ominous signs.[111]

A serious matter was raised by Urad-Nanaya in the spring of 670 BC (month of Iyyar). Although the letter itself includes some medical advice for the king, the first part of the letter concentrates on politics:

> Because of this speech of the king, Aššur and the great gods bound and handed over to the king these criminals who plotted against the (king's) goodness and who, having concluded the king's treaty together with his servants before Aššur and the great gods, broke the treaty. … (SAA 10 316)

Urad-Nanaya congratulates the king on arresting a group of "criminals" (*parriṣutê*) who "broke a treaty" which they had concluded with the king before Aššur and other state gods (SAA 10 316). But is this really a rebellion, and if so why would it concern Urad-Nanaya? The Chief Physician, judging by his letters, was an extremely sober and practical professional who hardly engaged in personal exchanges with the king, unlike his exorcist colleagues, who regularly complained to the king about very personal matters. Why would a physician comment on an internal criminal matter which had nothing to do with his duties as physician?

The political events mentioned in this letter concern Urad-Nanaya directly but have not been properly understood. All palace professionals had been required, two years earlier in 672 BC, to swear an oath of allegiance (*adû*) to the crown, and the list included every scribe (*ṭupšarru*), diviner (*bārû*), exorcist (*mašmaššu*), and augur (*dāgil iṣṣūri*, lit. "bird-watcher") (SAA 10 6 and 7). Furthermore, the "criminals" mentioned in Urad-Nanaya's letter were not criminals in the legal sense, but rather "cheats" or "quacks." The same word (*parriṣu*) was used by the court astrologer Nabû-ahhē-erība in a letter to the king in the very same year (670 BC), a few months later, in which the writer complained that an astrologer colleague supplied the king with wrong information about a sighting of Venus and what this would portend. Nabû-ahhē-erība pulls no punches, calling his rival a "lightweight," "fool," and "fraud" (*parriṣu*) (SAA 10 72: 9–10). In a similar fit of temper, Urad-Nanaya is actually complaining about his professional colleagues, whom he calls "frauds" or "quacks" (*parriṣutê*), who had sworn an oath of allegiance to the king but subsequently abrogated it by offering poor professional advice and service. Urad-Nanaya was not commenting in a casual way about contemporary politics, but he was accusing his professional rivals of incompetence and deceit.

Urad-Nanaya finally gets to the real point by reporting that he is sending the king some medicinal plants. In this regard, he was faced with the usual dilemma of physicians, whether to dazzle the patient with technical science or use layman's language to explain the treatment. Both approaches can be useful, and in fact Urad-Nanaya uses both. In this letter, he recommends the following drugs:

> The plants which I am sending to the king are the two which they call ᵘBU and ᵘ*Hat-ti*.[112] They do not resemble each other.
>
> The one which is like the base of a ring is heavy and very expensive. (SAA 10 316: 15–19)

Urad-Nanaya anticipates the king's obvious question, "what are they good for?", to which he provides the answer, that these plants are useful for counter-charms against witchcraft (*ušburrudû*) and specifically for women in labor (who especially required anti-witchcraft charms).

Neither plant can be found with these names in the medical corpus. Scribes required specialized training to read and write scientific literature, such as omens and medical texts, and it is doubtful whether the king himself would have understood the meaning of technical plant names. On the other hand, the purpose of the letter was to inform the king about a new drug, and a technical name did not need to be understood in order to make the desired impression. In fact, the name of the plant could be entirely bogus and still have the desired effect. The second plant, called ᵘ*Hatti* or "Hittite"-plant, could refer to a foreign plant brought from Syria, giving this plant exotic status. The description of this plant as having "the base of a ring" is unclear to us, but the fact that the plant was said to be "very expensive" or "very rare" (*uqur adanniš*) would not have escaped the king's approval. Recent research has shown that expensive placebos are more effective than cheap ones.[113] The point is that Urad-Nanaya does not expect the king to be familiar with the pharmacopeia, but he needs to impress upon Esarhaddon that he is prescribing new and exotic drugs to deal with the royal ailments, perhaps counting on the placebo effect of new drugs as well as any actual medical properties they may have possessed.

Since his royal patient suffered from a variety of chronic illnesses, Urad-Nanaya did not always take the same tack when offering medical advice to the king. For Esarhaddon's ear problems, he recommended the use of fumigation, which happens to be one of the most effective methods of introducing drugs into a patient's body, often being quicker than swallowing a substance. One of Urad-Nanaya's own medical tablets, copied by his disciple, contains a recipe for ear problems listing "9 drugs for fumigation of the ears" (see Geller 2007b: 13 and 18). In this particular case (SAA 10 323), Urad-Nanaya recommends two drugs, commonly used in medical ear-disease recipes, to be dripped into the ear. In his letter to Esarhaddon, Urad-Nanaya prescribes these drugs by their technical Sumerian names (^{šim}gig and $^{\text{šim.d}}$maš) rather than by their generic Akkadian terms, *kanaktu* and *nikiptu*, since these plants were well-known by their Akkadian names in non-medical usage as aromatics and hence may not have seemed like legitimate *materia medica*. Urad-Nanaya's own medical tablet for ear maladies employs these same drugs (Geller 2007b: 12, 70).[114]

We have some idea about Urad-Nanaya's pharmaceutical repertoire, since this cautious physician left us a list of drugs he used for fumigation, salves, and potions, mostly intended for diseases of the ears, although these same drugs could also be used for seizure (*saharšubbû*) and paralysis (*šimmatu*), since some drug preparations usually had multiple applications (SAA 10 327). Urad-Nanaya's list was his own inventory of what was available to treat conditions which were not easily treatable, such as a seizure, paralysis, aphasia, and ringing in the ears.

Urad-Nanaya labeled his drugs as *bulṭu, napšaltu,* and *nēpešu*, "recipe (or remedy), salve, and ritual" – three useful ways of categorizing the various uses for *materia medica*. Texts often refer to a *bulṭu latku*, "a tested recipe." The end product of the prescription is a potion, bandage, salve (as in this context), suppository, etc., but this is not sufficient. Many times recipes are accompanied by an incantation to be recited as well as a ritual to be performed. Each of these categories – recipes, ointments, and rituals – required its own brand of drugs.

Urad-Nanaya responds to the king's complaint about having a "fever"[115] by prescribing the rather simple solution of rubbing bird fat on the skin in order to protect the king from the effects of draughts, and when the king regularly washes his arms in the bath, the water should not be hot (SAA 10 318). There is nothing particularly remarkable about this recipe, since bird fat (usually referring to the fat of a goose) occurs in medical texts (Herrero 1984: 53), as does bathing in hot water (Herrero 1984: 97).

A letter from Urad-Nanaya to Esarhaddon dating from early 670 BC (SAA 10 315; Parpola 1983: 229) again refers to fever, this time as *hunṭu*, for which Urad-Nanaya prescribes a lotion (*marhuṣu*). Esarhaddon suffered from chronic fever, for which Urad-Nanaya struggled to find a remedy that would work and each time promised that the condition would abate. On the other hand, Urad-Nanaya's positive assessment of the effectiveness followed "best practice" as far as medical texts were concerned; conventional medical recipes always end with a final note that the "patient will get better" or "will improve." Nevertheless, he thought it best not to pull any punches with his royal patient by trying to promote his skills beyond what was possible to accomplish; Urad-Nanaya realized that chronic fever was not likely to be cured by the drugs at the disposal of a court physician. When asked face-to-face by Esarhaddon why he cannot find a correct diagnosis, Urad-Nanaya candidly replies that he cannot fathom the king's symptoms (*sakikkēšu*), and that the king could order diviners to check the omens to verify Urad-Nanaya's medical advice. The level of Esarhaddon's fever probably posed difficulties for Urad-Nanaya, and since there were no thermometers or instruments for taking precise measurements, Urad-Nanaya warns Esarhaddon that "perhaps the king will give off sweat" (SAA 10 315 reverse 14f.), indicating a high fever. On another occasion, Urad-Nanaya reported to Esarhaddon that one of his sons had periodically suffered from *hunṭu*-fever, but he reassures Esarhaddon that his son's "symptoms" are healthy.[116] We have no reason to believe that Urad-Nanaya was being overly optimistic in the latter case, since he seems to give sober assessments of medical conditions, at least as far as medical technique at the time would allow.

In the event, Urad-Nanaya also prescribes another type of treatment for Esarhaddon's fever, in this case a type of bandages called *ṣilbu* (pl. *ṣilbānu*), which probably gets its name from the criss-cross pattern of the bandages. Urad-Nanaya gives clear instructions for the application of these bandages: "just like they did it one or two times (before), let them apply them crosswise."[117] Urad-Nanaya even assures the king that he will come and "enlighten"[118] others as to the correct procedure for using these bandages; as Chief Physician, we can assume that Urad-Nanaya had a staff of other healers under his command.

Another letter of Urad-Nanaya refers to treating a skin lesion or scab (*sikru*) behind the ear in a young child of the palace (SAA 10 319). Urad-Nanaya writes that he applied a dressing and afterwards opened the bandage (lit. "rag," *širṭu*) and removed the pus, as much as on the tip of a small finger (see Parpola 1983: 252). Again Urad-Nanaya was following his own medical practices, as we can see from an Assyrian medical text which offers rich descriptions of pus (as well as blood or another fluid) flowing from a patient's ears, for which a tampon was a standard remedy; this particular tablet was copied by one of Urad-Nanaya's disciples (see Geller 2007b: 4 and 18). However, in his letter to the king Urad-Nanaya avoided all medical jargon but used layman's language when discussing the prescribed remedy. In any case, since technical language of medical texts would normally been written in Sumerian logograms, it is unlikely that anyone untrained in this literature would have been able to comprehend the obtuse terminology.

Urad-Nanaya also wrote to Esarhaddon about remedies for nosebleed (SAA 10 321), a condition also suffered by one of Esarhaddon's sons (SAA 10 324: 8–10). The medical intervention recommended was a tampon containing the seeds of the plant *maštakal*, a drug commonly used in many kinds of medical remedies. Urad-Nanaya wrote out the common Akkadian name of the drug rather than its Sumerian logogram (^{ú}in.nu.uš) by which it was usually known in the technical literature. The tampon was also to be mixed with the "blood" of cedar, to be wrapped in red wool (*tabrību*). The "blood" of cedar is another common ingredient in medical texts when dealing with ears, as can be seen again in one of Urad-Nanaya's own ear-ailment recipes, copied by his apprentice, recommending 15 plants which are to be wrapped into a tampon, sprinkled with "blood" of cedar, and put into the patient's ears (Geller 2007b: 18). Urad-Nanaya's letter prescribing a tampon against nosebleed for the prince is essentially the same as his medical recipe, but using a "simple" rather than "complex" drug formula to treat the ailment; in other words, in his letter Urad-Nanaya prescribes a single drug instead of a combination of 15 different ones for a tampon. This pattern is typical of medical court letters, which tend to refer to simple rather than compound drug remedies.

Within Babylonian medicine, a tampon was used for all kinds of ailments requiring insertion into some part of the anatomy, particularly ears, but also the vagina (Herrero 1984: 107), usually to staunch bleeding or pus. Urad-Nanaya used a type of "red wool" (*tabrību*) for his tampon, although the wool is much better known in medical texts by its Sumerian logogram, ^{síg}hé.me.da. Not only is Urad-Nanaya using layman's language, but he employed the Assyrian dialect word for "red wool," rather than the terms *nabāsu* or *tabarru* known from contemporary Babylonian dialects. The same is true of other expressions used by Urad-Nanaya, such as his instructions that one should wrap the *materia medica* into a tuft of wool (*nipšu*) (SAA 10 321 reverse 14), a term so far unattested in medicine.

One other ingredient mentioned by Urad-Nanaya was the use of the "dust of the crossroads" (SAA 10 321 reverse 6), which occurs fairly frequently in incantation rituals and represents as much magic as medicine (Geller 2000: 336). Urad-Nanaya also recommends reciting the appropriate incantation over the tampon before inserting it into the nostrils, reflecting contemporary medical practice. The grey area between magic and medicine is obvious from the physician's correspondence with Esarhaddon, since while advising Esarhaddon on his attacks of fever, Urad-Nanaya promises to send (in addition to a salve) a leather bag containing a phylactery, probably consisting of amulet stones (SAA 10 315 reverse 15–18). Such sacks of amuletic stones, strung on a string and hung around the patient's neck, are frequently prescribed to counteract the effect of psychological distress (see von Weiher 1983: 109–21), although Urad-Nanaya may have judged that Esarhaddon required treatment for his poor state of mind as well as for his fever. Even a physician like Galen was not occasionally averse to the use of amulets if it improved the patient's mental state (Nutton 2004: 268f.).

We can also detect a degree of professional rivalry in some of Urad-Nanaya's letters when commenting on treatment delivered by other practitioners. He complains, for instance, that others are treating with tampons "without knowing (what they are doing)" (SAA 10 322 reverse 8). Urad-Nanaya criticizes other practitioners for placing tampons against the nasal cartilage and failing to staunch the flow of blood; he explains that tampons must be placed at the nostril openings, which will cause shortness of breath but also stop the bleeding (SAA 10 322 reverse 14–17). Unfortunately, he does not specify whether an exorcist or another court physician was responsible for this malpractice. Urad-Nanaya's letter is a rare instance of an explanation of how medicine was administered, no doubt the kind of information learned at first hand as an apprentice physician.

Urad-Nanaya seems to be able to handle almost any type of medical problem that arose, including dentistry. He mentions that Esarhaddon had written to him about his teeth, to which he responded that there are "many cures for teeth," although without recommending anything specific (SAA 10 320 reverse 4–5). This information is useful because of the nature of "tooth-disease" recipes, which recommend substances like alum for treatment of the gums but at the same time rely upon the celebrated incantation of the "worm in the tooth" for dealing with other kinds of tooth problems (Collins 1999: 262f.; Foster 1993: ii 878). Nevertheless, tooth disease remained within the province of the *asû*, as Urad-Nanaya's letter indicates.

One wonders how a physician such as Urad-Nanaya spent his time. We can assume that he visited patients, since he continually reports on their state of health: "The king's son (enjoys) very good health. (When) I came to the king's son, he told me that 'all my body (lit. flesh) has improved'" (SAA 10 323: 7–11). According to the Diagnostic Handbook visiting the sick was the speciality of the ka.pirig-exorcist, not the physician, so the fact that Urad-Nanaya visits his patients may show how the theory was not always followed in practice. Otherwise, Urad-Nanaya makes one reference to his routine: "I am now busy cooking up (*materia medica*) in a (stone) *burallu*-vessel" (SAA 10 323 reverse 9–11), a type of cooking vessel otherwise unknown from medical texts. Urad-Nanaya was probably owning up to the fact that he spent a large part of his time making up recipes, in the capacity of *asû* as apothecary.

The concocting of recipes was not simply a manual activity of mixing ingredients but also involved keeping meticulous records, as Urad-Nanaya comments to Esarhaddon in a letter dated to June 669 BC, referring to purging a patient (perhaps the king himself): "In all recipes it is said as such: '(if) he purges (bile) through his mouth or his anus, he will get better'" (SAA 10 326 3′ – reverse 3′).[119] Although this quotation from the medical literature may have been intended to impress Esarhaddon with the writer's erudition, it also shows Urad-Nanaya's familiarity with current practices, since the citation occurs many times in medical texts dealing with rectal disease: "he purges through his anus, he will get better" (*BAM* 7 34: 50 and 37 ii 21′).[120]

It may have worried the Chief Physician that he was not unique in his professional judgment, since the Chief Exorcist, Adad-šumu-uṣur, offers nearly the same medical advice as Urad-Nanaya (SAA 10 217), at approximately the same time, in a letter to Esarhaddon (669 BC, around June), commenting about the king vomiting up bile. Adad-šumu-uṣur reports that the king's "natural state" (*šikinšu annû*) is not favorable, but after they "purged" the king "upward and downwards" (i.e. through mouth and anus) and induced sweating, he was better. The classic medical terms in which Adad-šumu-uṣur describes the treatment are difficult to differentiate from what Urad-Nanaya advises, and in fact Adad-šumu-uṣur may even be referring to the purging that was originally prescribed by Urad-Nanaya. The dates of the correspondence show that exorcist and physician were consulted at about the same time regarding the king's condition, and that both physician and exorcist were aware of the patient's recent medical history. The question is whether physician and exorcist were working in tandem or in competition with each other (see Jean 2006: 131–3).

Adad-šumu-uṣur was one of Esarhaddon's chief exorcists, whom the king consulted regularly about his own health and that of his family. In 672 BC Esarhaddon wrote to him, lamenting the death of one of his children, to which Adad-šumu-uṣur frankly replied, "If (the illness) could be resolved, you surely would have given up half of your lands if you had been able to resolve it" (SAA 10 187: 10–12). Adad-šumu-uṣur was not being philosophical in his reply but was, with some subtlety, absolving himself for the failure to cure the child, since his use of the word "you" ("if *you* had been able to resolve it") suggests that *someone else* had been responsible for the unsuccessful treatment.

This is not the only strictly medical matter brought to the exorcist Adad-šumu-uṣur. Like his colleague Urad-Nanaya, he visited the princes suffering from *hunṭu*-fever, since he reports in one letter that the prince is very well because "the fever has left him" (SAA 10 193: 7–8). Nevertheless, we must not exaggerate the "medical" aspects of Adad-šumu-uṣur's report on Assurbanipal's fever, since in the same letter he recommends that the king be subjected to the "substitute for Ereshkigal" ritual, a magical ritual reserved for serious cases of illness (SAA 10 193: 14).[121] This dramatic ritual involved wailing for the dead, who were already anticipating descending to the realm of Ereshkigal, goddess of the Netherworld, and it was likely to have been reserved for conditions deemed to be very grave. At sunset, the patient takes a virgin goat to bed with him and holds it in his lap. They then enter a room where the ground has been freshly dug, where both patient and goat are thrown to the ground. The patient's throat is touched by a wooden dagger, while the goat's throat is cut with a bronze (or copper) dagger. The inner and outer body of the goat is washed, anointed, and perfumed; it is dressed with clothes and even shoes of the patient, with *kohl* being applied to its eyes. The patient then gets up and leaves the room, with the exorcist (*mašmaššu*) reciting various incantations and mourning rites, declaring that the patient "has gone to his fate," i.e. died. Funerary rites are then carried out for the virgin goat, in place of the patient, and the goat is properly buried. The fact that Adad-šumu-uṣur recommended this kind of ritual for Assurbanipal (and not for his brother Šamaš-šuma-ukin) indicates the gravity of the *hunṭu*-fever and how non-medical therapies were employed side by side with drug therapy.

In this same way, Adad-šumu-uṣur sends three incantation tablets to the king (SAA 10 194 reverse 2′–6′), probably from his own library, which would have differed considerably from tablets sent by a physician. When the queen mother takes ill, Adad-šumu-uṣur recommends a group of 10 incantations with their appropriate rituals; these were designed to counteract the consequences of a bad omen (so-called *namburbî*-rituals) (SAA 10 201; see Parpola 1983: 148). In other letters Adad-šumu-uṣur refers only to rituals being performed, without their associated incantations, such as a ritual to counteract "weight loss" (SAA 10 200 reverse 5′ and 212: 12; Parpola 1983: 156), as well as general *ušburrudû* rituals against witchcraft, which incidentally had also been recommended by Urad-Nanaya on another occasion (SAA 10 200 reverse 6′).

On the whole, Adad-šumu-uṣur's advice given to Esarhaddon is not dissimilar from that of his physician colleague. He likewise advises the king against spending too much time in the dark (SAA 10 196: 14–reverse 6), probably to avoid being depressed. Furthermore, the exorcist advises the king about his diet and general behavior, by offering the following good advice: "being short of temper without eating or drinking disturbs the mind and illness results (lit. descends)" (SAA 10 196 reverse 15–18e). It seems that Adad-šumu-uṣur takes a somewhat different approach to that of Urad-Nanaya. While the physician concentrates on symptoms, the exorcist tries to look at the patient's behavior patterns, temperament, and diet, as a way of gauging his general health. We have no records of an actual diet or regime, except when ingesting drugs or when the physician occasionally advises the patient to reduce his intake of food and beer.

One of Adad-šumu-uṣur's most intriguing letters involves the testing of a new drug. He writes to Esarhaddon about a drug[122] which the king had previously asked about, and which the king himself claimed was "very good." Adad-šumu-uṣur suggests a kind of clinical trial: "Let us first have those slaves drink (it), and later let the princes drink (it)" (SAA 10 191: 11–13; Finet 1957: 137f.). At about this time, a formal oracular question was put to Šamaš by diviners during an extispicy, which was omens taken from the entrails of a ram. The question addressed to the Sun-god was whether the crown prince Assurbanipal was to drink a certain drug (SAA 4 187; Parpola 1983: 131). The diviner asks whether by drinking a particular drug Assurbanipal would be saved and get well. It is easy to imagine that the problem of Assurbanipal's health was of such severity that more than one type of practitioner was asked to intervene and do what he could. After the diviner presumably received a positive answer from the omens regarding the effectiveness of this drug, Adad-šumu-uṣur was also consulted and suggested testing the drug.[123]

The importance of Adad-šumu-uṣur's recommendation to have slaves try the drug is twofold. First, it appears to be a probable case of testing to see whether a drug works and what kind of pernicious side-effects it might produce. We have no way of knowing whether the slaves in this case suffered from a similar ailment as the crown prince or, more likely, were healthy guinea pigs. This letter may offer a clue as to how the effectiveness of a drug could be noted and perhaps even recorded for future reference. The second important aspect of the letter is that it is written by an exorcist rather than an *asû*-physician. The stereotypical image of the exorcist primarily concerned with incantations and spells rather than with prescribing drugs or recipes turns out, in practice, to be inadequate.

4

Medicine as Literature

Treating Babylonian medical texts as literature deserves special consideration. Like other literary compositions, medical texts or components of these texts exist in multiple copies, inviting comparison. Unlike other literary texts, however, medical texts combine prose and poetry, in which the recipes themselves are prose compositions, but frequently accompanied by poetic (even doggerel) incantations. Most but not all of Mesopotamian literature can be classified as poetry, but no other genre of literature quite compares with the mixture of prose and poetry that one finds in the Babylonian medical corpus.

Three main types of medical texts constitute distinct literary genres. We have already encountered prognostic omens of the Diagnostic Handbook (Labat 1951; Heeßel 2000), with its listing of symptoms from head to foot from various "diseases." A second type consists of lists of plants and stones used as *materia medica* (see Schuster-Brandis 2008), or lists of diseases, usually belonging to the scholastic curriculum. A good example of this genre belonged to one Nabû-ile'i, an apprentice *asû* from Assur from a known family of scribes, and the inventory itself is designated as belonging to *asûtu* (*BAM* 1 1). The great majority of medical texts, however, consists of therapeutic texts containing a mixture of recipes, lists of *materia medica*, and incantations. These can either be small single-prescription tablets or large compendia, in which recipes are marked off by rulings, and groups of recipes intended for the same ailment are given, with the first entry giving the full symptoms, and subsequent entries just having "ditto."

Diagnostic Handbook

The Diagnostic Handbook is a good place to begin, from a genre viewpoint. Actually, the Diagnostic Handbook has been widely misunderstood as referring to patients, when in fact it really refers to disease and to patients only as carriers of disease. It is worth emphasizing that this work is not a list of case histories of individual patients, but rather a list of how diseases show up in patients within set patterns that can be recognized and recorded. We have no idea how many observations of how many different patients have produced these symptoms, since each line of text may well represent symptoms drawn from a multitude of patients.[124]

Although understood as diagnostic omens, the language and vocabulary of the Diagnostic Handbook hardly resemble those of other omen compendia. There is no real similarity either in language or contents, except for the general syntactical format of protasis and apodosis clauses. One might imagine, on the contrary, that the listings of symptoms in medical diagnostic omens would closely match descriptions of similar symptoms for the same ailments within the therapeutic texts. Stol has found some parallels (Stol 1991–2), but surprisingly few, when the entire corpus is taken into account (see also Kinnier Wilson and Reynolds 2007). In most cases, symptoms described in the Diagnostic Handbook use a much different language to that found in the therapeutic texts to describe the same disease and symptoms.

Here is an example from a prescription:

> [If] his urine is like ass urine, that man suffers from "discharge."
> [If] his urine is like beer dregs, that man suffers from "discharge."
> [If] his urine is like wine dregs, that man suffers from "discharge."
> [If] his urine is like clear paint, that man suffers from "discharge."
> If his urine is like *kasû*-juice, that man is overcome by "sun-light" disease.
> If his urine is yellow-green, that man [suffers] from stricture of the groin.
> If his urine is white and thick, that man [suffers] from a dissolving calculus.
> If his urine is like *dušû*-stone, that man [suffers] from a calculus.
> If his urine is as normal, but his groin and epigastrium cause [him] pain, that man suffers from stricture of the rectum (var. bladder). (*BAM* 7 5: 1–10)

Contrast this passage with a similar passage from the Diagnostic Handbook, describing the very same symptoms of the color of the urine in kidney disease:

> [If] his [urine] is red, it is the hand of his god, (his disease) will be prolonged; if his urine is yellow, [his] disease will be [prolonged; ditto, he is affected by sun-fever, he will die].
> [If] his [urine] is black, he is affected by the fatal disease, he will die; if his urine is dark, [he will die].
> [If] his urine is continually blocked up, he will die; if his urine keeps flowing, [he will die].
> [If] his urine and his sperm keep flowing, he will die; if his urine is [....] like [..., he will die].
> [If] his urine is like water, his illness will be protracted, but he will recover; if his urine is like pitch, [ditto].
> [If] his urine is like wine, his illness will be severe but he will get better; if his urine is like milk, [he will recover].
> [If] his urine is normal, ditto.
> [If] his urine is inspected and produces a fleshy-membrane, (the patient) was attacked from the steppe (i.e. by a demon).
> [If] his urine is inspected and produces his actual flesh, he was attacked in the steppe. (*BAM* 7 49: 14′–22′)

The basic differences in these descriptions suggest that therapeutic recipes and diagnostic omens were composed in different scribal "workshops."

Medical Incantations

We can readily appreciate why incantations would be used with magical rituals, since they are essentially dramatic affairs intended to impress the patient with elaborate and powerfully moving spectacles: fumigations, peeling onions and wiping the patient with flour, massage, scapegoat rituals, drum-beating, and other kinds of rituals (which we might consider as hocus-pocus). Medicine was, on the whole, much more subdued: the patient was treated with potions, suppositories, oiled reeds inserted into his penis, bandages, and amulet stones hung around his neck, as well as the occasional incantation. There is, however, a grey area between these two spheres of influence, consisting of incantations exclusively applied to Babylonian therapeutic prescriptions.

Incantations within medical recipes form a genre of their own. There is little point in trying to deduce worthy medical information from the incantations themselves, as if medical incantations had some particular role to play within diagnoses and treatment (Collins 1999: 64–122;

Geller 2007a: 390, 396). On the contrary, the incantations within the medical corpus tend to be rather jejeune and simplistic, many with abracadabra-type formulae, more akin to nursery rhymes than sophisticated magic.

Several incantations are situated within medical prescriptions for eye disease to treat cloudy vision, filmy eyes, eyes filled with blood, and so forth. One incantation within this corpus alludes to the dangers of surgery:

> Incantation. Eyes with the porous blood-vessel, why have you been blurred by chaff,
> thorns, *šuršurru*-fruit, or river algae (var. algae tossed up by the river)?
> Why have you been blurred by clods in the streets or twigs in *recesses*?
> Rain down here like a star,
> keep falling here like a meteor, before the flint(-knife) and scalpel of Gula reach you.
> An irreversible incantation, the incantation of Asalluhi-Marduk and the incantation of Ningirimma, master of spells,
> and Gula, master of healing arts, has cast (it) and I have taken (it) up.
> Incantation spell.
>
> ---
>
> Incantation for removing chaff, twigs and whatever from the eyes.
>
> ---
>
> (*BAM* 510 174–80)

The point of this incantation is that blurred vision can be caused by various types of foreign objects in the eye, such as algae from the river, debris of plants, or dirt from the street. "Raining down" is probably a reference to tears washing out the intrusive objects, and the spell makes a threat: the foreign matter must leave the eye as soon as possible, with the speed of a falling star, or else the patient will be subjected to the surgeon's scalpel. The actual phrase used, "scalpel of Gula," is meant as an oblique warning that the sick eye had better heal itself before it requires the doctor's intervention. Since Gula was the patron goddess of *asûtu* (see Figure 4.1), we can guess that a physician's scalpel is alluded to in this incantation, although we have no independent evidence to confirm that the *asû* acted as a surgeon.

The healing goddess Gula and her son Damu make frequent appearances in medical incantations, but often in a rather practical mode. The following incantation occurs within the same collection:

> Incantation. The open eye is open, the open eye is open, the angry eye is angry, the open eye is angry,

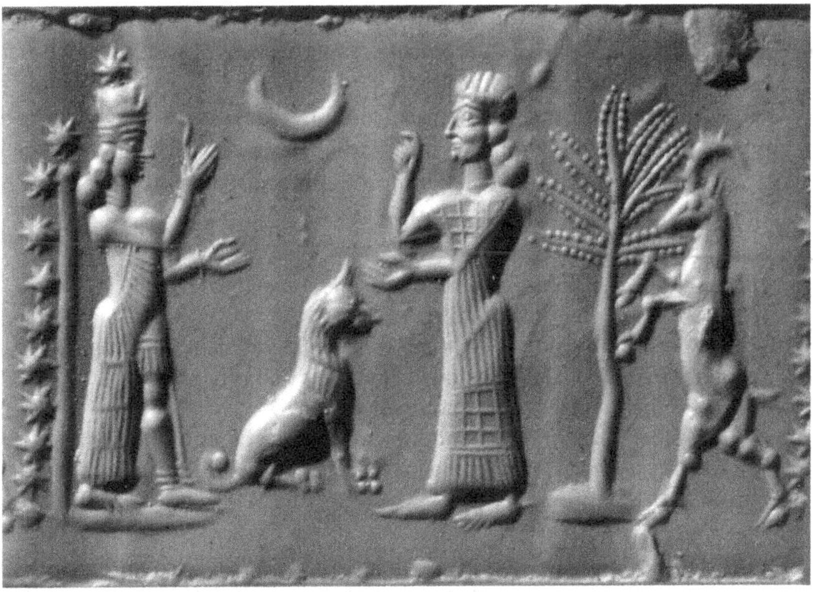

Figure 4.1 Healing goddess Gula with her dog, holding a scalpel in her right hand and a tablet in her left hand (Collon 1987: No. 793; photo courtesy D. Collon)

> the look is *crouching*, the look is evil, thick eyes, cloudy eyes,
> porous [in (its) veins], the eye *pissing* blood like the sacrifice of a male sheep.
> (The eye) is (affected by) "shadow-disease" like the water floating with the swamp and seaweed, like the vinegar floating in the jug.
> A mud-wall is built between them (the eyes), Nergal entered and his seat[125] is placed in between,
> because of this "seat" within that one, preventing breathing
> freely. The incantation is not mine, it (belongs to) Ea and Asalluhi,
> the incantation (belongs to) Damu and Gula, the incantation (belongs to) Ningirimma, mistress of incantations. O Gula – heal and receive your fee.
> Incantation spell. (*BAM* 510 84–90)

It is the last line which engages our interest, since it repeats a phrase found frequently in medical incantations, asking Gula to heal the patient and to take her fee. The fact that this is a "fee" rather than a "gift" (as usually translated) can be seen from a late Uruk incantation which spells it out unmistakably. In this text the healer tells the patient that he deserves to be healed since "you have given a fee to the exorcist" (von Weiher 1983: No. 22, 113), and the patient afterwards declares before the god Šamaš, "I gave a fee to your servant, the *mašmaššu*-exorcist, in front of you."[126] Since the exorcist was an active priest in the temple, such a gift for services rendered makes good sense, and what we have here is a polite reminder that healing costs money.

The following brief incantation from the same text is a mixture of simple Sumerian logograms and Akkadian phrases, with some levels of meaning which we cannot fully comprehend, comparing the eye ailments to a storm:

> Incantation. The open eye looks, the open eye sees, the cloudy eye is clouded, the open eye is clouded.
> The two eyes are sisters in between which a mountain is put across,
> above them a knot is tied, below them a clay wall is built.
> Which is their wind, which is not their wind?
> Which is the onset of their wind, which is not the onset of their wind?
> The storm ahead is dark, the surface of the pupil [of the eye is dark]. (*BAM* 510 121–6)

The image is clear: the two eyes are sisters, and the nose and mouth are described as a mountain and clay wall, from which wind emanates; these images may be based upon a doll or figurine. "Wind" is often a disease agent in medical texts, either as a draught or flatulence. The poem otherwise tells us little about the disease itself or its causes, but there may be a teleological image referring back to creation, judging by another incantation from the same eye-disease text:

> Incantation. In the beginning before creation, the "water-carrier" (*alalu*) came down to earth,
> the seeder-plow bore the furrow and the furrow
> the shoot, the shoot the seedling, the seedling the node, the node the ear of barley, the ear of barley
> the stye (in the eye). Šamaš gleaned and Sin gathered, and while Šamaš was gleaning and Sin gathering,
> the stye entered the lad's eye. Attend, Šamaš and Sin, and let the stye go out. [Incantation spell].
>
> ---
>
> Incantation for removing a stye from the eyes.
>
> ---
>
> (*BAM* 510 181–6)

Eye disease, in this case caused by an insect or something very small, originates from time immemorial when agriculture was first established (see Collins 1999: 95f.; Foster 1993: ii 854). According to the ontology of this incantation, agriculture led to disease in humans, and even beneficial activities such as sowing and reaping had harmful results, but no specific information given is relevant to actual diagnosis or treatment.

One very short incantation in this group poses the simple question asked by every patient: "Why me?"

> [Incantation.] The veiled eyes, the confused eyes (with) porous blood vessels, [the] two (eyes) cry towards their mother Mami:
> "Why (does it happen) to us and (why) did you saddle us with *ašû*-disease, blood, and wind?" Incantation spell. (*BAM* 510 163–5)

One distinction between magic and medicine is how each approach deals with the patient's personal trauma. The question "Why me?" is not likely to be answered by the *asû*, and the patient would probably be advised to go and ask the exorcist.

As mentioned, one of the main features of formal magical incantations is a bilingual Sumerian-Akkadian format, usually referring to a dialogue between Marduk and his father Ea. One incantation within the same group of eye-disease medical recipes is a bilingual Sumerian-Akkadian medical incantation, which resembles (in form at least) incantations from the realm of magic, as if borrowed from a *mašmaššu*-colleague:

> Incantation. The wind was blowing in heaven and a sore settled in a man's eye.
> It blew iṇ from the distant heavens (Sum. and a sore settled in a man's eye.)
> A sore was found in the sick eyes.
> The eyes of that man are troubled, his eyes are blurred,
> and when by himself that man cries bitterly.
> Nammu (var. Nāru) noticed that man's illness:
> "Take crushed (var. cooked) *kasû*,
> recite the Eridu incantation,
> bind the eye of that man."
> When Nammu (var. Nāru) touches the man's eye with her pure hand,
> may the wind which is swept into a man's eye be removed from his eye. (*BAM* 510 151–61)

This incantation has some hallmarks of a formal bilingual incantation of a *mašmaššu*-exorcist. Instead of a dialogue, however, between Marduk and Ea, the protagonist is the goddess Nammu, Ea's mother, who appears in other incantations as patron goddess of the Apsû, the subterranean sweet waters. In this role, Nammu acts like Marduk: she "notices" the man's illness and has to decide what is to be done, although she has no one to whom to turn for advice. These conventions are quite rigid and cannot be easily altered by whoever composed the incantation.

There is an anomaly here, since an earlier version of this incantation from Sultantepe[127] has the river god Nāru appearing in place of Nammu in later versions. The river god Nāru was elsewhere invoked in *namburbî* incantations to counteract evil portents because the river carries off the bad magic which had been tossed away (Maul 1994: 85–9). Nāru also appears in hemerologies, schedules of lucky and unlucky days in the month; if you asked Nāru the river god a question on a certain day of the year, he would answer you with "news" (Labat 1939: 98f.). But mostly Nāru is associated with the River Ordeal, in which the innocent man is thrown into the river and survives but the guilty is drowned, with his recovered body covered with sores and bleeding from his orifices; it is the god Nāru who does the judging, one presumes, but our information is far from abundant (see Lambert 1965: 6, 9). In any case, the older variant from Sultantepe with the river god Nāru does not conform to the usual tropes of exorcistic incantations,[128] and the later version of the incantation makes the goddess Nammu (rather than Nāru) protagonist, perhaps because the incantation places the spell within the city of Eridu, Nammu's residence and gateway to the Apsû. Nammu notices the patient's sore eyes and takes some remedial action, and that is about it. This medical incantation appears to have been altered to look like standard exorcism, but in fact it is far less elaborate than conventional incantations emanating from the exorcist's workshop.[129] Moreover, these medical incantations are not overly theological in trying to pin the cause of disease on sin and transgression (see van der Toorn 1985: 76). According to them, disease just happens.

There are some exceptions to this pattern. Medical texts dealing with childbirth contain rather more elaborate incantations, comparing the fetus to a boat on the water and the mother giving birth to the Cow of Sin, the moon god (Stol 2000: 64–70). We also find the familiar formal dialogue between Marduk and Ea, suggesting that these incantations were composed by an exorcist, rather than as an afterthought of an *asû*-physician. These childbirth incantations within the medical corpus are exceptional, but childbirth is exceptional, for several good reasons. Childbirth is not a disease, it concerns women not men, and it can need serious magic to help it along. In some sense, childbirth medical texts may be considered as more conservative than other types of medical texts, but, if so, Babylonia is not alone in this. Within the Hippocratic corpus, the treatise dealing with diseases of women is also considered to be more conservative than other treatises, containing more elaborate pharmacological recipes and exotic ingredients (Nutton 2004: 98).

An incantation is primarily an encounter between forces which try either to harm or to protect mankind. Malevolent forces can be anything from an evil demon to an evil or angry god, witchcraft, bad omens, envy (described as an evil eye or evil tongue), negative effects of violating a taboo, or just plain bad luck, and divine powers can be marshaled to help, as we know. The real subject of the incantation is usually the human victim. Is it the same in medicine? The simple answer is "No." The Diagnostic Handbook consists of long lists of symptoms drawn from patients, organized from head to foot, drawn from all kinds of diseases and affecting every part of the body – but we have no idea how many patients were behind each symptom. Ten? A hundred? The least likely possibility is that each symptom represents an individual case from a single patient. The same is true of the therapeutic medical recipes, which never refer to any specific patient by name or otherwise, and it seems obvious that these are not case histories. Recipes are aimed at a disease or diseases of any number of patients which share the same symptoms and signs.

This may ultimately explain why the medical corpus includes simple incantations, to give the impression that gods also maintain an active interest in the patient's well-being and health. Introducing incantations into medical texts may have been an attempt to make the medicine somewhat more personal. On the other hand, the last thing a physician wants is to be confused with an exorcist.

Therapeutic Prescriptions as Genre

A typical feature of medical texts shows duplication most often occurring with individual recipes, drawn from different contexts, rather than whole compositions being duplicated. In fact, the process of duplicating passages within Babylonian therapeutic texts is unique, when compared to other types of cuneiform literature. The usual pattern, outside of medicine, is for a composition to exist in various manuscripts, which are mostly the same or similar. Incantations are a good example. Entire tablets and compositions appear in multiple copies, normally with variants among manuscripts. Not so with medical texts; often a single line of text, representing a single recipe, may be duplicated between one text and another, but within completely different medical contexts. We will see how this works.

Therapeutic texts are normally constructed from individual recipes or prescriptions, and each individual medical recipe therefore had a semi-autonomous status and could be cited freely between different genres of therapeutic texts. We do not understand the system behind these citations, but texts dealing with one medical condition might quote a recipe designated for a different ailment altogether.

Let us look at a typical example. The following text is from seventh century BC Assur, from the private house of exorcists, which contained a considerable medical library as well as texts relevant to magic and exorcism (Maul 2004: 81f.), and it has duplicates from the Nineveh state library founded by Assurbanipal.

1 [If a man] suffers [from discharge], crush together *kukru*, *ata'išu*,
2 myrrh, and alum,
3 and he drinks it in strong wine on an empty stomach.

---

4 If ditto, "silver-lustre"-plant, *puquttu* seed,
5 *pallišu*-plant/stone, *sāpinu*, (var. *azallû*-seed), *baluhhu*-resin,
6 ["donkey]-vulva"(-shell), shell of ostrich-egg,
7 myrrh, coral; (total) 9 drugs
8 for discharge, checked, he keeps drinking it in wine.

---

9 If ditto, "pure"-plant, "mole-cricket," *kukru*, *šunû*,
10 madder, myrrh, *baluhhu*-resin,
11 *šunû* seed, *taramuš* seed, *ṣumlalu*,
12 fat, and almond(wood); [crush] together these 11 drugs
13 and boil them in ghee, his thighs
14 (and) his buttocks [..............

Reverse

1′–2′ ....
3′ put [............] into it and pour it into his penis.

4′ If ditto, *urnû*, ditto, ditto, ditto.

5′ [If di]tto, crush fox-vine, ditto, ditto, ditto.
6′ pea, myrrh, and horned alkali,
7′ coral, alum; 5 drugs.
8′ If a man repeatedly rises[130] because of his urine,
9′ he keeps drinking (the drugs) either in beer or in wine or water.

10′ Crush together *imhur-lim*, myrrh, ostrich-egg shell,
11′ black frit, for 3 days in fish brine,
12′ for 2 days in drawn wine, and for 3 days in

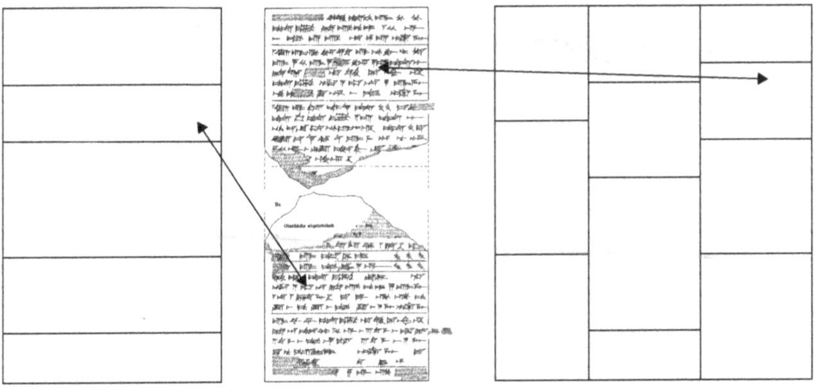

Assur plant list (*BAM* 164) Assur recipes (*BAM* 116) Nineveh plant list (*BAM* 431)

Figure 4.2 Assur recipes *BAM* 116 and duplicate recipes (*Babylonisch-assyrische Medizin*)

13′ pomegranate-juice, and he keeps drinking it
14′ [for a] stricture of *midday*.

15′ Hurriedly excerpted for his [lecture] (colophon). (*BAM* 7 7)

The recipe concerns kidney ailments. Other texts duplicate no more than a single recipe from this composition, consisting of only a few lines. Two of the partial duplicates from Assur are lists of medicinal plants which include a section of drugs specifically for kidney disease. As for the *materia medica* it is likely that the medical recipe and lists drew upon some common source.

The great Nineveh library provides another example of a kidney disease text (see Figure 4.3), but only two lines of the Nineveh text duplicate the Assur text above (*BAM* 116):

> Its ritual (dù.dù.bi): Crush together *imhur-lim*, myrrh, ostrich-egg shell, black frit, for 3 days in fish brine,
> for 3 days in drawn wine, and for 3 days in pomegranate-juice, he keeps drinking it and he will improve. (*BAM* 7 2 ii 19–20)

What is unusual is that the Nineveh text writes dù.dù.bi "its ritual," to introduce these two lines; this type of dù.dù.bi rubric usually introduces an exorcistic ritual which follows an incantation (Herrero 1984: 26), and in fact these two lines immediately follow an incantation in the Nineveh tablet (*BAM* 7 2 ii 18). In other words, the same therapeutic recipe in an Assur tablet is employed as a "ritual" and follows an incantation in a Nineveh tablet.

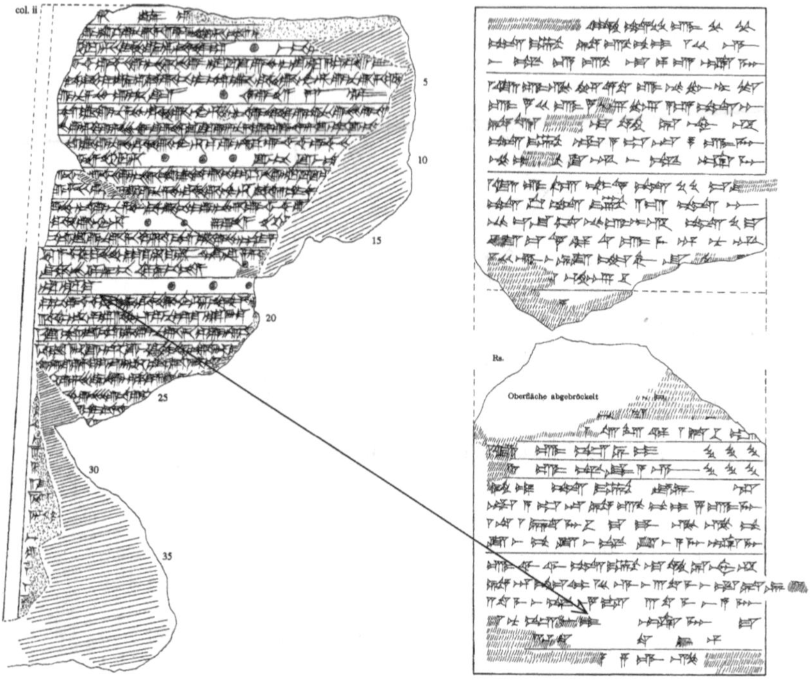

BAM 7 Nineveh

BAM 116 Assur

Figure 4.3 Duplicate recipes (*Babylonisch-assyrische Medizin*)

If we compare the contexts of these two tablets, we can see that both recipes from Assur and Nineveh were used within medical compositions to combat kidney disease. The Assur tablet is a single-column tablet and its contents, according to the colophon, were "hastily excerpted," either for a lecture or for application. The tablet contains various recipes which could have been drawn from a longer composition, while the Nineveh tablet is a multi-column library composition with many recipes against kidney ailments. We have two completely different genres of texts, one from Nineveh being a major compendium of medicine, the second from Assur being a teaching tool in which a few important or typical recipes have been excerpted and compiled. There is little otherwise in common between these tablets. Are these the same literary genre? I think not, because a library reference work is quite different from a textbook or digest of texts for pedagogic purposes. Tablets could be excerpted for a variety of reasons. For instance, another Assur tablet composed by the well-known Assur exorcist Kiṣir-Nabû introduces a recipe for making an ointment for the anus and claims to have excerpted the recipe from many different sources and collected the information together into a single tablet; the colophon explains that this excerpt was made hastily for the purposes of performing a specific medical treatment (*BAM* 7 42); the tablet is excerpted *ana ṣabat epēši*, "for use." This kind of tablet should also be differentiated from a standard library reference work.[131]

Another example of two different genres of medical texts which share common recipes occurs in recipes for a diseased anus, which also contain prescriptions employed in tablets dealing with "cough" (*suālu*). The precise medical connection between rectal ailments and "cough" (which could include diphtheria or pneumonia) is unclear. The following text is a case in point.

–1 If a man's limbs are *poured out*, his chest and shoulders hurt him,
0 his arms, shins [and knees] hurt him, his testicle, either on the right side or on the left,
1′ bothers him, and he shows blood in his urethra, that man
2′ suffers from stricture of the anus. To cure him, you heat in an oven (l. 9) *taramuš*, *imhur-lim*,
3′ *kukru*, [...........], juniper, *suādu*,
4′ sweet reed, *ballukku*, *šimeššalû*,
5′ cedar, *šupuhru*-cedar, *šunû*,
6′ *urnû*, *hašû*, *nuhurtu*,
7′ *nīnû*, dates, malt-flour, beer,
8′ wine-drops, ...-barley.
9′ You pour (it) into the anus.

10′ [If a man] suffers from rectal disease and his anus stings him,
11′ mix [together] juniper, *kukru*, *ṣumlalû*, [and .....]
12′ [pour] *kanaktu* and a clump of malt in oil and beer into his anus.

13′ If a man suffers from a sore anus and has piercing pain
14′ and his belly cannot take in food and fluids (and) pours out mucous from his anus,
15′ to cure him: pour *hašû* (and) *urnû* in *kasû*-juice
16′ into his anus.

17′ If a man's bowels are bloated, his intestines
18′ make a lot of noise like (that) of an *išqippu*-bird,
19′ that man suffers from flatulence and "sun-fever".
20′ His condition is of long duration, (it is) the Hand of the Ghost; in order to cure him, heat in premium beer (l. 24) *nīnû*,
21′ "mountain"-plant (*azupīru*), *hašû*, *nuhurtu*,

22′ juniper, *kukru*, *ṣumlalû*, *ballukku*,
23′ *cuttings of* aromatics, field-clod, – 11 plants,
24′ filter and cool them, add oil into the (mixture),
25′ pour it into his anus and he will recover. (*BAM* 88 = *BAM* 7 27)

These lines come from a single-column tablet (provenance unknown) dealing with rectal problems. The prescriptions in this tablet were known both in Assur and Nineveh, since they occur in no less than seven other manuscripts representing three different genres of medical texts. Let us describe a few of the other manuscripts. Two tablets (*BAM* 52 and 168) belong to the same prolific Assur scribe, Kiṣir-Nabû, and both probably come from the Exorcists' House in Assur. The colophons of both tablets explain that these manuscripts consisted of excerpts hastily made for treatment or pedagogic purposes (see Hunger 1968: No. 212); the colophon of one of the tablets, mostly devoted to diseases caused by cough (*suālu*), specifies that the tablet was a "sixth excerpt of a collection of (medical) recipes, based upon a wax tablet from Assur, the original being from Uruk, written and checked" (*BAM* 52). Another tablet owned by the scholar Kiṣir-Nabû contains recipes from diseases caused by the Hand of the Ghost (a common cause of illnesses), as well as kidney and anal disease recipes (*BAM* 7 34). A third duplicate comes from Nineveh, a four-column library tablet devoted mostly to diseases also caused by the Hand of a Ghost (*BAM* 471). All of these texts have different orientations and purposes within their own specific contexts.

One manuscript mentioned above deserves a closer look, and we offer below a selection of recipes from this prescription (*BAM* 168):

18 If a man suffers from "sun-fever," flatulence, paralysis, lameness, *šaššaṭu*-disease,
19 Hand of the Ghost(-disease), Hand of the Oath, disease of the rectum, (or) any disease, in order to cure him,
20 10 shekels of "health"-plant, 10 shekels of *tiātu*, 10 shekels of *ata'išu*,
21 10 shekels of *hašû*, 10 shekels of *nuhurtu*, 10 shekels *nīnû*,
22 10 shekels of *urnû*, 10 shekels of clump of salt, 10 shekels of *azupīru*,
23 10 shekels of *šibburratu*, 10 shekels of "white" plant, 10 shekels of alum,
24 10 shekels of juniper, 10 shekels of *kukru*, 10 shekels of *aktam*, 10 shekels of salt,
25 10 shekels of madder seed, 10 shekels of *ṣumlalû*, 10 shekels of *suādu*,
26 10 shekels of *baluhhu*, 10 shekels of cedar, 10 shekels of myrrh,
27 10 shekels of "sweet reed," 5 shekels of *sihu*, 5 shekels of *argannu*,
28 5 shekels of *barīrātu*, 5 shekels of "sun"-plant: pound and sieve these 25 drugs
29 and aromatics together. Take premium beer, *kasû*-juice

30 and strong vinegar, add this powder (of ground up ingredients) to it,
31 heat (it) in an oven, take it out in the morning, cool (it), add honey and pressed oil to it,
32 pour (it) once, twice, and three times into his anus.

---

45 If a man suffers from stricture of bladder, 2 shekels of myrrh, 2 shekels of *baluhhu*-resin,
46 juice of *hašû*, juice of *nuhurtu*, salt-water, the juice of all of these aromatics:
47 take a half sila of each of these juices, pound them together, boil (it),
48 you filter (it), cool (it), mix a half (sila) of oil with them. Crush 7 grains of "health"-plant,
49 add (it) into (the mixture), divide the fluids into 3 parts and
50 pour (it) into his anus once, twice, and three times, to relieve his constipation (lit. to cause the stopping up of his bowel to pass through).
51 If *uršu*-sores are smashed (or) if the hemorrhoids are plucked off,
52 the illness will be relieved, his anus will be widened; this lotion
53 (is) for releasing from an oath (and) for all kinds of disease.

---

66 If a man's bowels need to relieve constipation (lit. cause a stoppage to pass) or crush sores and pluck out hemorrhoids,
67 weigh out juniper, *kukru*, *nuhurtu*, horned alkali, "health"-plant,
68 in equal measure, boil (them) in beer or vinegar, you filter it,
69 cool it, put oil into it (var. honey or oil), pour (it) into his anus.

---

70 If a man's groin hurts him at an inappropriate time, and his shins
71 cause him a stinging pain (var. he stretches out his feet), he is weak in his thighs and his knees (var. shins) gnaw at him with pain (var. are cold for him),
72 that man suffers in the rectum (already) during his youth. To cure him:
73 crush in equal amounts black *kamūnu*, *nīnû*, *kanaktu*, "health"-plant,
74 *kasû*, mix them in fat and make a suppository,
75 sprinkle (on it) cypress oil, insert it into his anus and he will improve.

---

76 If ditto, bat guano, *nīnû*, *baluhhu*-resin, "white" plant,
77 dates (var. of Dilmun), gourmet-salt, ox fat, these 7 (var. 6) drugs for a *powerful* suppository.

---

78 You dry out Dilmun dates, horned alkali, fat of the kidney of a male sheep,
79 *kukru*, juniper, *ṣumlalû*, *baluhhu*-resin,
80 *abukkatu*-resin – 8 drugs – insert a suppository
81 into his anus to stop flatulence; a proven remedy (var. a proven suppository which stops wind).

---

82 Kiṣir-Nabû son of Šamaš-ibni hastily excerpted (this) for application. (*BAM* 7 34)

Here we see a text covering a variety of different medical problems, and the colophon explains that these recipes have been hastily extracted for treatment (*ana ṣabat epēši*, "for use").[132] One of the recipes gives amounts of drugs (either five- or ten-shekel amounts) for general conditions: fever, flatulence, rectal disease, several kinds of paralysis, and two categories of disease known by theoretical causes (Hand of the Ghost and Hand of the Oath[133] diseases), or simply used as a panacea ("any disease"). Another recipe in this collection describes an elaborate enema for bladder ailments (stricture). Further recipes refer generally to bowel problems and hemorrhoids, and some of these prescriptions are older and already attested at Sultantepe, an eighth-century library found in modern Turkey. Every recipe in this Kiṣir-Nabû excerpt tablet has a duplicate from some other manuscript, which is not always the case with medical texts.[134]

Sometimes we find a tablet containing unique medical prescriptions (i.e. no duplicates found as yet), but the tablet will also include a recipe which appears in many other manuscripts. For example, one Assur text with relatively few duplicated passages (*BAM* 104) has one line (l. 34) which occurs in three other manuscripts. One of these duplicates (*BAM* 152) is a four-column tablet containing recipes for ailments of the head, feet, and rectum. A second duplicate (*BAM* 95) is written in a "landscape" format (with the longer side being its width rather than height), and may represent an older text tradition, while the third duplicate from Sultantepe[135] certainly goes back to an older eighth-century text tradition (see Figure 4.4).[136]

Let us return to the question of why the same drugs would be used within two different genres of medical texts, having entirely different medical uses and aims, for entirely different parts of the human body or organs. Two possibilities come to mind. One, recipes were associated with each other as literary compositions and learned as such, and hence recipes which were thematically related (e.g. referring to diseases of the rectum) would often be copied together in the same sequence in different tablets. For example consider the following three recipes:

> If a man's limbs are flaccid (lit. poured out), his chest and shoulders hurt him,
> his arms, shins [and knees] hurt him, his testicle, either on the right side or on the left,
> bothers him, and he shows blood in his urethra, that man suffers from stricture of the anus.
> To cure him, you heat in an oven (l. 7) *taramuš*, *imhur-lim*, juniper, *suādu*, sweet reed, *ballukku*, *šimeššalû*, [cedar], *šupuhru*-cedar, *šunû*, *urnû*, *hašû*,

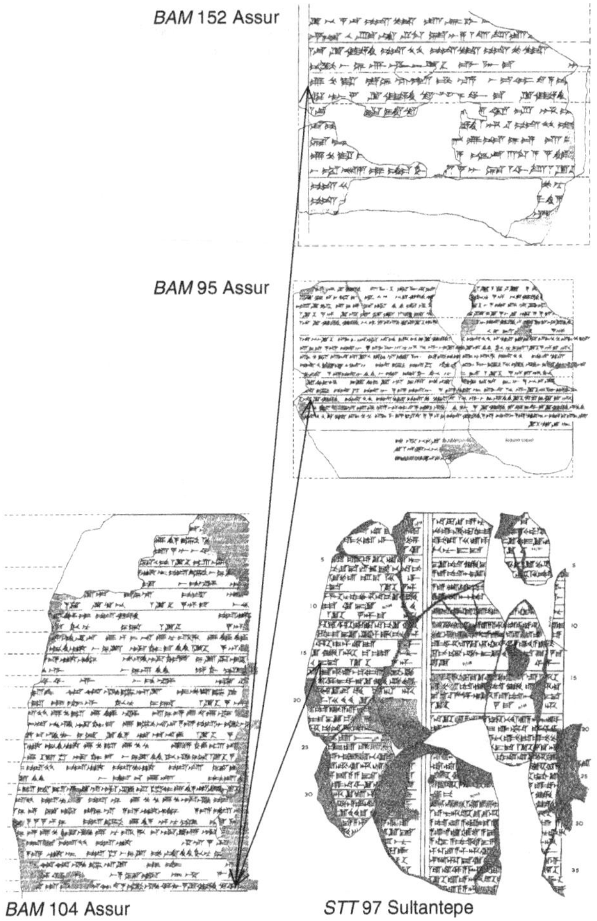

Figure 4.4 *BAM* 104 and duplicates (*Babylonisch-assyrische Medizin*)

nuhurtu, *nīnû*, dates, malt-flour, beer, wine-drops(?),
and …-barley, and you pour (it) into the anus.

If a man suffers from rectal disease and his anus stings him and his bowels are cramped and he is constipated,
boil vinegar and premium beer, cool it and pour it into his anus.

[If a man] suffers from rectal disease (and) it stings him: mix together juniper, *kukru*, *ṣumlalû*, [.….
<boil> *kanaktu* (and) clump of malt in oil and beer and [pour it] into his anus. (*BAM* 7 32 1–11)

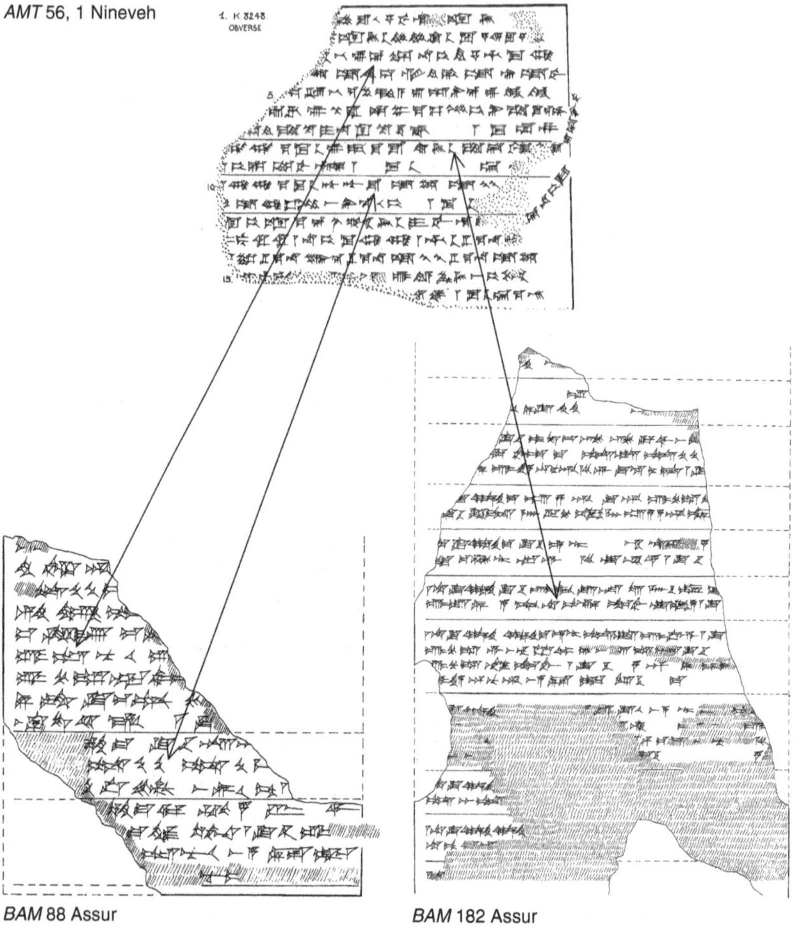

Figure 4.5 *AMT* 56,1 and duplicates *(Assyrian Medical Texts* and *Babylonisch-assyrische Medizin)*

The recipes above come from a Nineveh manuscript (*AMT* 56,1), a single-column tablet (hence probably not a library tablet), written in Babylonian script,[137] which has recipes for rectal disease on the obverse and recipes for stiffness in hips and groin on the reverse. This Nineveh text has several duplicates for these lines, two of which are from Assur, both dealing with rectal disease (*BAM* 88 and *BAM* 182).

The Assur recipes duplicate the Nineveh recipe in the same sequence, but with one important difference: another two-line recipe intervenes (see Figure 4.5).

> If a man is ill in the rectum and his anus stings him and his innards are bloated, he suffers from constipation; boil vinegar and premium beer, cool (it) and pour it into his anus. (*BAM* 7 32 8–9)

It is difficult to discover whether any literary scheme lies behind these complex arrangements.

This pattern repeats itself throughout Babylonian therapeutic medical literature, with one important exception: eye-disease texts. The British Museum houses a collection of three lengthy Nineveh tablets devoted to eye disease, and these tablets are unusual in being three complete manuscripts of the same therapeutic text (*BAM* 510, 513, and 514). It is not easy to know why eye texts were copied as complete manuscripts while other recipe collections were not, but, nevertheless, the composition is in fact more complicated. These Nineveh tablets contain only a couple of individual recipes also attested elsewhere, but these same few duplicated lines appear in no less than three other Assur tablets.[138] When we finally find a duplicated eye recipe, it turns out to be popular, also known in Assur. An exceptional text from mid-first-millennium BC Sippar provides excerpts from a variety of medical texts dealing with many different conditions, but two lines of this text also duplicate a single recipe in the Nineveh eye-disease manuscripts (see Heeßel and al-Rawi 2003: ii 15–19). It is strange that this is the same recipe duplicated in Assur. Hence, a single three-line recipe in a large Nineveh medical eye-disease text appears in various Assur medical sources and a Sippar school compendium, but few other duplicated passages are to be found. It is difficult to explain this pattern.

A different scenario appears in another Assur tablet from the Louvre dealing with ear disease (Geller 2007b), copied by an apprentice of Urad-Nanaya, the senior court physician at Assur. Many of its lines are also duplicated on the same Sippar extract tablet mentioned above (Heeßel and al-Rawi 2003), as well as duplicated recipes in other Assur tablets and tablets from Nineveh, Babylon, Uruk, and Nimrud, showing how widely popular individual recipes might be. It should not be surprising that prescriptions for ear symptoms employ the same recipes as tablets devoted to the disease caused by the Hand of the Ghost, since the disease was often thought to be caused by a ghost whispering into the patient's ear (Scurlock 2006: 14). This kind of association of ideas can partially explain how similar recipes can appear in different medical contexts. However, recipes may have been copied in several manuscripts with more regard to literary composition than to medical efficacy. Recipes often (but not always) occur in the same general sequence, even if another recipe intervenes.

The literary character of recipes can also be seen within the listing of *materia medica*, since plants and stones are often given in standard sequences, which were learned by the medical scribes (Tavernier 2008: 193f.). It is unlikely that we will find a medical reason for *materia medica* to be listed in a fixed sequence within recipes, other than that scribes found it easier to remember ingredients in this way.

Poetry Within Therapeutic Prescriptions

The idea that medical recipes could be composed in poetic form rather than prose might seem alien to a modern reader, but such texts were well known in the classical world. A second-century BC priest of Apollo and physician from Claros in Asia Minor, one Nicander, composed a lengthy Greek remedy in 958 lines of hexameter verse against venomous creatures and their bites. His work was called *Theriaka*, the name later given to a recipe popular in the Roman world as an antidote and later general panacea (Watson 1966: 13 f.).

Despite the lack of evidence for poetic recipes in Babylonian therapy, medical texts are not entirely devoid of poetry. Incantations serve as the poetic component of therapeutic texts. Medical incantations are poetic and often revolve around literary themes which have little specific application to the recipes. The passage below, for instance, shows recipes phrased in the second person in the form of instructions for treatment, while the interspersed incantations are in the first person singular, as abbreviated passages containing allusions to more cosmic motifs. The medical incantations themselves provide a literary structure which aims to define the role of the practitioner as a powerful figure, well connected with the powers governing heaven and earth.

> If a man suffers from *maškadu*, he must keep drinking (from a potion) gourd, *e'ru*-seed, and *kazallu*, [crush] "field-clod"-plant, "scorpion"-plant. (Then) mix flour in premium beer, and when you make a concoction, [he will improve].

....

> Incantation. I impregnate myself, I impregnate my body, just as a dog and bitch or pig and sow
> have had sex in the steppe; just as a plough has seeded the earth and the earth has received its [seed],
> so I cast the spell that I receive (it) in myself and in my body,
> and impregnate himself (and) [his] body and [cause the evil to depart].

Incantation for *maškadu.*

(*BAM* 7 31: 11′ 13′; 18′–21′)

A somewhat different view of medical incantations is provided by an Assur text, *KAR* 73, now *BAM* 7 9–10 (see Böck 2008: 307f.). This single-column tablet contains two poetic incantations, with one medical extract between them sufficient to show that the context is medicine, not magic. The format of the tablet is unusual, since the incantation on the obverse is ruled while that on the reverse is not.[139] We give the reverse here only, since the obverse, although an incantation, is essentially a hymn to the healing goddess, Gula.

1 When (it is the case): if a man (suffers from) either *pardannu* or *sahhihu*-disease,
2 discharge or stricture or a rectal disease,
3 he constantly has dripping urine,
4 as if being struck down by a weapon – like a (menstruating) woman –
5 or whatever other illness which is not recognized,
6–7 its remedy (lit. ritual): you sprinkle pure juices of juniper in front of Gula, you set up a *small* altar, on a roof, the place of ritual preparation,
8 (on which) you sprinkle dates and *sasqû*-flour, you place *mirsu*-cakes of honey and butter,
9 you set up an *adagurru*-vessel (and) you either make a pure offering or a *prayer*.
10 You set (on the altar) the shoulder, the fatty meat and the roast-meat,
11 crush together *hašû, ata'išu*, sweet-plant, "single"-plant, *šumuttu, sahlû*,
12 and put (them) into premium beer, and place it before Gula.
13 Have the patient kneel and you *fumigate* your hand over him,
14 you withdraw and that patient raises up in [his] hand the premium beer which you set out and he recites thus:

15′ Incantation. I beheld your face, [O Gula], august healer,
16′ [..........], you are supreme and pre-eminent (var. the pure one),
17′ I beheld this drug which I hold up before you.
18′ On this very day, (the patient) has either *pardannu* or *šahhihu*-diseases,
19′ either discharge (var. or stricture) or rectal disease or loin disease, or dribbling of urine, or one is struck by a weapon like a (menstruating) woman, or whatever illness with which I am sick,
20′ and you know what I do not know: am I to drink this drug?
21′ With these drugs let me be healthy, let me be well, let me be happy,
22′ so that I may praise your great divinity! [Incantation spell.]
23′ "In every corner let them bless Gula,

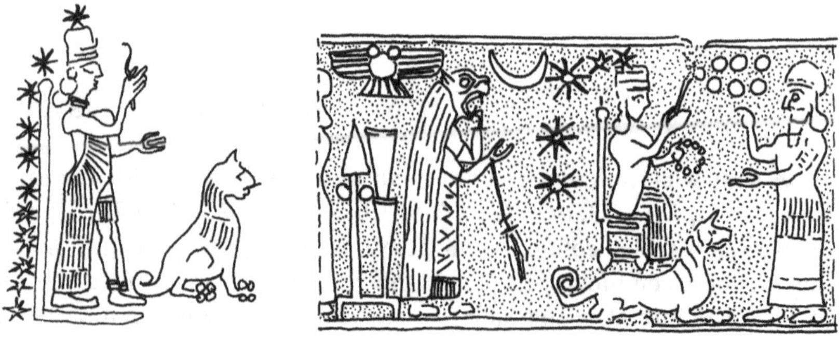

Figure 4.6 Healing goddess Gula with her dog, seated before the god Latarak (R. Ellis, Fs. J. J. Finkelstein, figure no. 3; drawing F. A. M. Wiggermann)

24′ who is supreme in spells and healing,
25′ great is her medicine, Gula heals those who revere her.
26′ By the command of Baba I will praise and call her name to everyone,
27′ when I go before her." Three times you will have him recite it (the incantation) and he will bow down,
28′ he will drink this drug and bow down, and recite thusly:
29′ "I drank this healing drug of my goddess,
30′ [..] and I was cured." He says this three times and bows down.
31′ [........] he keeps drinking this drug and he will recover.

Again we note the characteristic first-person-singular orientation of the incantations, expressing the healer's special relationship with the goddess of healing arts, Gula, while the therapeutic recipe takes the usual form of second-person instructions for treating the patient. Within the incantation, the patient is referred to in the third person, as if a character in a drama, while the incantation priest asks rhetorical questions about the effectiveness of the cure (but always anticipating a positive reply).

This is not to suggest that medical incantations have a fixed format or structure, since there is a great variety of themes expressed within them. In a Nineveh medical text which is partially duplicated in Uruk, one incantation is devoted to *būšānu*-disease, which affects the nose and mouth:

> Incantation. *Būšānu*, strong is his grip, it seized the uvula like a lion,
> it has seized *soft tissue* like a wolf, it has seized the *tender part*, it has seized the tongue,
> its "seat"[140] is positioned in the windpipe(s). Go out, *būšānu,* not to be seized by you,
> like death which shows the way [a one-way voyage], or a stillborn child which cannot seize its mother's breast (var. milk),

> you must not return to what was seized by you. The incantation is not mine, it belongs to Ea and Asalluhi,
> the incantation of Damu and Gula, of Ningirimma, mistress of incantations, Gula, life-giving mistress,
> Gula *who makes life secure*, take your "gift" (i.e. fee). Incantation-spell.
> (Hunger 1976: Nos. 52 and 54, 55–61)

This incantation ends with the conventional formulaic lines explaining that the incantation belongs to the gods, not to the credit of the healer himself, since it would have been considered hubris for the healer to claim that the healing power comes from his own personal charisma. The healer himself was an instrument of the magic, but not the power behind it. The incantation itself provides some interesting and even important information, but within a magical framework which has little relevance to the therapies employed. The significant point is that the illness, in this case *būšānu*, has a "seat" or "topos" within the windpipe, which is the organ associated with the disease. The theoretical notion of the "seat" of a disease is expressed within the incantation because there is little scope for a therapeutic recipe to explain the thinking or theoretical basis behind the medicine. Medical incantations provided a mechanism for expressing more general ideas about the nature of healing and disease.

An obvious classification of medical texts differentiates between single recipes or prescriptions, usually on single-column or small tablets, and multi-column tablets containing numerous recipes, rubrics, and incantations. One assumes that the difference denotes individual prescriptions written out by the physician himself for the patient, as opposed to textbook or reference works in which many recipes are collected and recorded, perhaps taken from tablets containing a single recipe. As for single-column tablets containing relatively simple texts, late examples from Achaemenid Babylon exhibit a consistent alternating pattern of medical recipes and incantations being written in either vertical or horizontal (i.e. portrait or landscape) formats; tablets with a portrait (vertical) orientation tend to be *asûtu* while those with a landscape (horizontal) orientation are *āšipūtu* (Finkel 2000: 146). This shows clear distinctions being made within late scribal schools between the physical shape of tablets dealing with medicine (*asûtu*) and those dealing with magical arts (*āšipūtu*). Scribes had to learn to write both. Nevertheless, it is not possible to prove that these single tablets were collected and copied into larger compositions.

A clear distinction can also be seen between medical recipes which give the amounts of each ingredient to be used, and those which do not. This is distinct from dosage, which is rarely specified. It may be that weights of *materia medica* (typically one or two shekels of each ingredient, or fractions thereof), reflect a more precise genre of medical practice, which attempts to calibrate the amount of each ingredient (see Finkel 2000: 146f.). The argument against this assumption is that, in most cases, the amounts given are standardized, so that the same amount (e.g. one shekel) of each drug is prescribed, which makes little sense in reality. One would hardly expect this in either a cooking or medical recipe, since the values and effects of individual ingredients are very different from each other.[141]

It is more likely, however, that recipes are schematic. Some weights and measures might be mentioned in order to give the recipe more authority, or to distinguish a medical recipe from a list of commonplace foodstuffs. We find this difference in later systems of medicine, such as in Maimonides' *Regimen for Health*, in which he lists foods which people ought to eat to maintain good health, but when Maimonides lists similar ingredients to be used as a drug, he usually specifies the precise amount of each ingredient to be used in the recipe. There are clearly different genres here: recipes without amounts and those with amounts.

The following treatment for kidney disease is an example of a recipe with weights of *materia medica* (*BAM* 7 9; Böck 2008: 311ff.). The recipe consists of a long list of 33 drugs, each beginning with the amount of 2 shekels, in three columns:[142]

2 shekels of *puquttu*, 2 shekels of *azallu*, 2 shekels of "dog's-tongue" plant
2 shekels of fox-vine, 2 shekels of raisins, 2 shekels of *šibburatu*-plant
2 shekels of cucumber, 2 shekels of gherkin, 2 shekels of ....
2 shekels of madder, 2 shekels of *aktam*, 2 shekels of *nuhurtu*-plant seeds,
2 shekels of root of male mandrake, 2 shekels of *pig-fat* plant,[143] 2 shekels of *kukru*,
2 shekels of juniper, 2 shekels of *ṣumlalû*-plant, 2 shekels of *šimeššalû*,[144]
2 shekels of *abukkatu*-plant resin, 2 shekels of *suādu*, 2 shekels of myrrh,
2 shekels of male *nikiptu*, 2 shekels of female *nikiptu*, 2 shekels of ....
2 shekels of *azupīru*, 2 shekels of *šumuttu*, 2 shekels of....
2 shekels of *samīdu*, 2 shekels of "detox" plant,[145] 2 shekels of ....
2 shekels of *nitku*, 2 shekels of .....
2 shekels of peas, 2 shekels of lentils, 2 shekels of .....
2 shekels of madder, 2 shekels of pomegranate, 2 shekels of ...
2 shekels of *e'ru*-wood, 2 shekels of .... 2 shekels of .....
2 shekels of *šunû*, 2 shekels of *alamâ*,[146] 2 shekels of *kamantu*,
2 shekels of coral, 2 shekels of sea-pebble, 2 shekels of sea-....,
2 shekels of sea-stylus, 2 shekels of "donkey-vulva" shell, 2 shekels of yellow ochre,

2 shekels of *kalgukku*, 2 shekels of *muṣu*-stone, 2 shekels of loadstone,
2 shekels of *zalaqu*-stone, 2 shekels of frit, 2 shekels of black frit,
2 shekels of *ṣumlalû*, 2 shekels of *pallišu*-stone, 2 shekels of *sāpinu*-stone,
2 shekels of *alluharu*, 2 shekels of *qitmu*, 2 shekels of alum,
2 shekels of pumice, 2 shekels of kak.na$_4$, 2 shekels of ostrich-egg shell,
2 shekels of block salt, 2 shekels of red salt, 2 shekels of steamed salt, variant: half a shekel of each of the salts.
Total of 9[4] drugs soaked for "stricture."

There are two other drug-inventory tablets from Nineveh, probably from the same archive, which give the same listing of drugs and have the same rubric, "in all: 94 drugs, these to be soaked."[147] In the Nineveh inventories, *only* the drugs used against kidney-disease are listed with their two-shekel weights (as in the text above); no other drugs in the lengthy inventories have associated measures.

What do we make of a list of ingredients duplicated in very different texts (one a medical recipe and the other an inventory of medicinal plants), but both extracts having the same format? Can we call this a literary convention ("two shekels" plus drug) or is there something special about this particular group of drugs used against kidney ailments? Variant readings within texts can also point to readings based upon literary rather than medical considerations. The final line of a kidney-disease recipe reads, "½ shekel of block salt, ½ shekel of red salt, ½ shekel of steamed salt" (*BAM* 7 11: 34′). This line relates to a final phrase in a similar recipe which reads, "2 shekels of block salt, 2 shekels of red salt, 2 shekels of steamed salt, variant: ½ shekel [of each of] the salts" (*BAM* 7 9 32f.). It is likely that the latter scribe was working from two sources, and that the variant was more literary than medical.

Occasionally medical texts give listed weights in fractions of a shekel, such as "handfuls" (*BAM* 7 16). Other texts have various weights of ingredients, as one might expect, as in the following extract from what can be considered an ancient Physician's Desk Reference text:[148]

1 Two shekels *kukru*, two shekels …
2 two shekels *ballukku*, half shekel *juniper*,
3 two shekels fine reed, one shekel [drawn] vine,
4 half shekel *ata'išu*, one shekel *raisin*,
5 half shekel *mint*,
6 half shekel *būšānu*-plant
7 one shekel *imhur-lim*-plant, one shekel *imhur-ešra*-plant
8 two shekels cucumber, (all of which) you heat in beer.

9 You (then) put oil and honey into it, [knead it] into a powder.
10–12 This lotion is effective and tested against jaundice and hepatitis.
13 Lotion of oils (for) "sun-fever." (*BAM* 186)

The colophon of the tablet tells us that this tablet belongs to Mr Kiṣir-Assur, exorcist (*mašmaššu*) of Assur, and that the recipe was "hastily extracted for a use in a treatment."

Other examples of Babylonian recipes list minute amounts of drug weights, such as eye salve prescriptions giving amounts as an eighth of a shekel (*bitqu*), 15 "grains" (= a twelfth of a shekel), and a twenty-fourth of a shekel (von Weiher 1983: No. 50).

Such Akkadian recipes have equivalents from the Greco-Roman world, such as a recipe for the "windpipe" recorded by the Roman physician Celsus in the first century AD:

> 4 grams each of Cassia, iris, cinnamon, nard, myrrh, frankincense
> 1 gram of saffron,
> 30 peppercorns boiled in 1½ liters of raisin wine until the consistency of honey. (Celsus [Loeb], 2 5 25)

Note how the major ingredients all share the same amounts (4 grams). Compare this with a Greek recipe against gout and sciatica, attributed to Proclus, which looks altogether too schematic:

> 9 ounces of germander
> 8 ounces of centaury
> 7 ounces of birth-wort
> 6 ounces of geniat
> 5 ounces of *huperikon*
> 4 ounces of Macedonian parsley
> 3 ounces of *meon*
> 2 ounces of *agarikon*
> 1 ounce of *phou*
> 2 kotylae of Attic honey. (Tecusan 2004: 623)

The question is whether these amounts were real or imaginary, in all our ancient medical sources.

The Babylonian Background to Greco-Roman Pharmacology

In 66 BC the Roman world was transformed by the news of the defeat of King Mithridates of Pontus, but the effects of this victory were further reaching than could have been anticipated. According to accounts preserved by both Pliny and Galen, Mithridates had perfected an antidote against poison, and it proved to be so effective that he was unable to poison himself after his defeat but had to be killed by a soldier. The Romans found an entire library with recipes, and the Roman Lenaeus was ordered by Pompey to translate and copy the recipes for Rome. Although Lenaeus' work does not survive, there are reports that the Mithridates antidote or theriac caused a sensation in Rome because, as Pliny remarks, plants had not been studied by Roman physicians. Although not the first recipe of its kind, the Mithridates antidote was widely quoted as a compound recipe against venoms (a theriac) and poisons, and even as a general panacea; it became popular among drug-sellers throughout the Empire (Watson 1966: 81).

The question is why the Mithridates antidote became so popular in Rome, since similar preparations had been known to Greco-Roman medicine for centuries. Antiochus III of Mesopotamia, for instance, was reported to have developed a theriac against venoms already in the second century BC, which consisted entirely of herbs and may have relied upon more ancient Babylonian sources; other theriacs were known from further west (Watson 1966: 13). There are several factors, however, which may have influenced the reputation of the Mithridates antidote. One is that we are not told in which language the recipes were written, although scholars assume them to have been composed in Greek. Nevertheless, Pontus was located in the Orient, in Asia Minor, and the recipes may have been based upon a much older tradition of medicine (in the local language?) than that preserved in Greek, similar to the theriac of Antiochus III. Another factor is the information that Mithridates had first tried out his antidote on criminals; records of such experimentation are rare.[149] Finally, the Mithridates antidote became famous as a panacea partly because it was a compound recipe consisting of some 90 ingredients, while in Greco-Roman medicine it was often the practice to rely upon *pharmaka* or "simple" drugs, i.e. single drugs employed against single conditions.

A famous example of a theriac was recorded by the first-century AD Roman Celsus, ascribed to Mithridates. The recipe reads as follows:

1.66 grams of costmary
20 grams of sweet flag
8 grams each of hypericum, gum, sagapenum, acacia juice, Illyrian iris, cardamom
12 grams of anise
16 grams each of Gallic nard, gentian root, dried rose leaves etc. (Celsus [Loeb], 2 5 23; see Watson 1966: 5–6)

We see in this compound recipe that although some ingredients appear in various amounts, other ingredients with identical measured amounts are grouped together. The same pattern can be seen in Babylonian medical texts specifying amounts of ingredients (see above).

As to why the Mithridates antidote became so popular, we need to examine the state of healing arts within the broader reaches of the Roman Empire as well as among its immediate neighbors, particularly in Mesopotamia, to gauge the proper medical context of theriacs and antidotes. In order to do this effectively, it is necessary to consider *systems* of medicine in the ancient world, rather than writings of individual physicians. We propose some general comparisons between so-called Hippocratic medicine and Babylonian medicine, although recognizing many sub-divisions within these two general categories of approaches to healing.[150] Essentially, Babylonian medicine was an extremely conservative system of healing, already well-established by the early second millennium BC, consisting of recipes and drugs used to treat diseases which were identified by careful examination and documentation of all external bodily symptoms as well as urine and other indicators of bodily functions. Disease was considered to be the result of external attack on the body, either by demons, or from natural causes such as bites, draughts, or poisoned food. The earliest phases of healing arts in Greece were probably very similar, as can be seen from early treatises within the Hippocratic corpus, which relied upon careful scrutiny of external symptoms. As in Babylonia, early Greek medicine expressed prognosis in the form of signs and omens, as indications of whether the patient was likely to live or die or survive for a limited time. Like Babylonian medicine, pre-Hippocratic medicine (referred to by the Hippocratics as *hoi archaoi* – the "ancients") considered disease to be the result of demonic attack, which often called for magical means to counteract it. Finally, like Babylonian physicians, Hippocratic physicians had only a rather vague idea of internal anatomy because few physicians conducted autopsies on human corpses (see von Staden 1998).

Hippocratic medicine as a general system departed from traditional Babylonian medicine in the fifth century BC by developing a new approach to both diagnosis and therapy. The primary notion of external attack by demons was replaced by the theory of humors or internal balance/imbalance within the human body, which had to be corrected through the use of diet, purgatives, and eventually minor surgery in the form of venesection. Writers usually consider Greek medicine to be more "scientific" than its Babylonian counterpart, in the same way that Greek mathematics improved upon that of its predecessors. In a comparable way, once a theory of humors was developed to explain all manner of disease, the practitioner could dispense with a cumbersome system of preparing prescriptions which had to be tailored to each individual condition and ailment. In other words, the simple rule replaces the exhaustive database. Although not necessarily more effective for the patient, the new Hippocratic methodology took its place among other emerging disciplines in Greek science, as begun by Thales and his contemporaries.[151]

5

Medicine and Philosophy

According to legends about Hippocrates, which no one takes seriously, he destroyed the medical archives of his rivals from the mainland city of Cnidos (or, alternatively, he destroyed all the medical books on his own island of Cos [Temkin 1995: 54]). The fact that alternative versions of this story were reported about Hippocrates may tell us something about his reputation, if not his life. The impression persisted among later Greeks that Hippocrates was an iconoclast who not only forcefully broke with his medical predecessors, but took active steps to destroy their work and methods. In some sense, he succeeded admirably. Hippocrates' innovations were aimed against a rival system or at least an older system of healing arts, which resembled Babylonian medicine in many respects. In the older strata of the corpus, pre-Hippocratic medicine was usually seen as being either old-fashioned or archaic. The precursors of Hippocratic medicine certainly lack the hallmarks of Greek medicine, such as a theory of humors, a focus on diet,[152] and minor forms of surgery (see Geller 2007: 191–3). In other words, pre-Hippocratic medicine from Greece comprised a *system* which most closely resembled that which we know from Babylonia. This system is characterized by very large collections of hundreds of plants and drugs, forming the basis for therapeutic recipes. Symptoms were also painstakingly collected from head to foot, although the derived insights were expressed as omens predicting whether the patient would live or die.

One of the noticeable differences between Hippocratic and Babylonian medicine is the lack of cuneiform texts dealing with diet and regimen. While Greek medicine invested a great deal of interest in diet and exercise and ways to preserve good health, Babylonian medicine was primarily focused on how to treat or alleviate symptoms and distress caused by an already existing ailment; little attention was paid in medical texts to prevention.[153] Disease can either be physical or psychic, and in ancient Babylonia could express itself through symptoms such as pain and fever and loss of appetite, or through anxiety, insomnia, impotence, or other "maladies d'esprit." While apotropaic magic may have been used to keep demons at bay, no medical recipes were designed to promote healthy living or prevent disease from occurring.

This cultural contrast ignores the much more complex relationship between "medicine" and "magic" which existed in Babylonia but also persisted within the Greco-Roman world as well. It is true that Babylonian medicine incorporated demons and incantations which we usually consider to be "magic." Nevertheless, the pattern of magical and medical texts within Babylonia generally shows two complementary approaches to healing. We have some long and complex compilations of incantations aimed at either avoiding or treating the attack of demons or ghosts or witchcraft or diseases, resulting from cultic guilt or divine wrath. On the other hand, the oldest medical text which we possess, in Sumerian, gives recipes without a single reference to either demons or incantations. Later Babylonian medical recipes deal with diseases and symptoms without necessarily referring to divine wrath, guilt, or demons, although incantations are often included among the recipes. The precise relationship between medicine and magic in Babylonia remains thorny and complicated.

The same, however, could be said of Greek medicine. The advent of Hippocrates and Hippocratic medicine in no way displaced belief in gods, demons, and the supernatural as components of Greek medicine. The popularity of the healing god Asclepius is one indication of the prominence of religion in therapy, as best exemplified by the popularity of his temples in the Greek world, even on Cos itself. The many dedicatory inscriptions from these temples offering thanks for healing are not the only evidence for belief in magical forms of healing; stories abound in Greek and in other languages about great charismatic healers who could heal through a word or by applying spittle to a patient. Apollonius of Tyana serves as a good example of a "wonder-healer" whose very touch had healing properties, and there seemed to be no shortage of adherents in the ancient world. Tatian, an "Assyrian" living in Rome in the second century AD, complains about popular belief in illness demons and the use of amulets against them, and he even argues against the use of drugs (*pharmakeia*) against illnesses, confirming that such notions were current at the time in the Greek-speaking world (Tatian [Loeb]: 33, 16–18). This is hardly the attitude inherited from Hippocratic medicine, but most probably reflected much of popular belief at the time, even if not shared by practitioners of medicine for the upper social classes, which forms the bulk of our medical literature.

Within Greek medicine, the role of the philosopher is thought be unique and entirely consistent with the emergence of Greek science. Hippocrates' contemporary Democritus claimed that "the medical arts heal diseases of the body, whereas wisdom relieves the soul of passions" (Temkin 1995: 8; see Edelstein 1967: 349–66). This distinction between physician and philosopher was reiterated by Aristotle, and Galen also remarks that "it is for [the philosophers] to shape the health of the soul itself because of something that is greater, whereas it is for the physician to do on behalf of the body, lest it easily slip into disease" (Temkin 1995: 14). These statements, emanating as they do from the perspective of Greek science, recognize tension between philosopher and physician, but at the same time ignore the competition for the patient's soul offered by Asclepius cults or charismatic healers in the Greco-Roman world who relied upon magic and incantations. It is this dichotomy between treating the soul and treating the body which interests us, since a similar dichotomy exists within Babylonian medicine and a similar tension between those who healed the mind and those who healed the body.[154]

The comparative paradigm is by no means perfect. Babylonians had no concept of the "soul" in the Greek sense, and the very idea of a Babylonian "philosopher" seems like an oxymoron. Although Babylonians aspired to wisdom and learning, including astronomy, medicine, mathematics, lexicography, and grammar, and even natural science in the forms of descriptions of stone and plants, this is hardly to be construed as contemplative philosophy. Even if late period texts in Babylonia could be shown to embody abstract ideas or observations, if not hypotheses, we would still hesitate to call it "philosophy," that quintessentially Greek pursuit.

There is no Akkadian word for "philosophy," nor does any other Semitic language have a "lover of wisdom." The concept of wisdom (Akk. *ihzu*)[155] does exist, and the closest equivalent phrase in Akkadian to "philosopher" is *bēl nēmeqi*, "master of wisdom," a title applied to the god Marduk but never to any mortal scholar or savant. Within the Babylonian *Weltanschauung*, only a god could be a real "master of wisdom," since no human could attain to such intellectual heights. In fact, not only is the god Marduk *bēl nēmeqi*, "master of wisdom," but he is also *bēl šipti*, "master of exorcism" *par excellence*. This accords well with the general idea of healing in Babylonia, since the exorcist never puts himself forward as a charismatic healer in his own right, but views himself solely as representative of Marduk, sent by Marduk himself as his agent. In Babylonia, gods heal and man is only the conduit. Man possesses knowledge, gods possess wisdom.

One other potential candidate in Babylonia for a "lover of wisdom" was the *apkallu* or primordial sage, with whom the exorcist identified in order to establish his prestige and *gravitas*. The *apkallu*, however, was an icon, an antediluvian figure who would have been comparable in the Middle Ages to a patron saint of exorcism, but even in Hellenistic Babylonia the *apkallu* was never envisaged as a philosopher.

There is an alternative approach to this notion of philosophers healing the soul and physicians healing the body. Several famous Babylon scholars in antiquity, known especially from colophons of tablets dealing with Babylonian "sciences" (astronomy, divination, and magic) might be considered as Babylonian "philosophers." One is the famous scribe Esagil-kīn-apli who is thought to have lived in the eleventh century BC, but whose contribution continued to be recognized by scholars even in the Seleucid period (Finkel 1988: 143ff.). He was not only a priest but remembered as a "scholar" (*ummânu*) who was credited with having compiled editions of loosely connected compositions dealing with the arts of the exorcist, such as diagnostic omens, physiognomic omens, and an assortment of all the major magical texts.[156] Esagil-kīn-apli's range of expertise also included medical and therapeutic texts which we would usually associate with the physician rather than the exorcist, and he is claimed to have been the author of an exorcism manual, a single tablet which lists incantations and medical texts by their incipits (Jean 2006: 73–4), as a catalogue of all major texts relevant to the training of an exorcist. Unfortunately, we do not know very much about how a Babylonian *ummânu* taught and how he explained difficult texts to his students; there was no doubt more abstract or theoretical speculation going on in the scribal curriculum than we are informed about.

The second Mesopotamian savant who appears frequently in colophons was something of a specialist in divination. Nabû-zukup-kēnu flourished in Assyria in the second half of the eighth century BC, and his forte was astronomy and astrology, judging by colophons on tablets. His tablet archive included multiple copies of astronomical omens and terrestrial omens, works on augury and oracles, and a copy of the Gilgamesh epic. His *oeuvres* also included several tablets of esoteric hermeneutics (Frahm 1999: 79). There is no doubt about the considerable learning and enormous spectrum of expertise commanded by Nabû-zukup-kēnu, but one would hardly refer to him as a philosopher.

Another candidate for Babylonian "philosopher" may be the Assur exorcist Kiṣir-Assur, who owned a considerable library of cuneiform tablets in the seventh century BC dealing with magic and healing arts, as well as esoteric wisdom. The range of subjects is again very impressive, judging by the tablets actually excavated from the house (Maul 2004: 79–96; Pedersén 1986: 44f.; Livingstone 1986: 260). Aside from the impressive collections of incantations of all types (including *namburbî*-omens and incantation rituals), Kiṣir-Assur's private library contained many examples of medical prescriptions. Like his predecessor Esagil-kīn-apli, there is no doubt that Kiṣir-Assur was an "exorcist" rather than "physician," judging by his title (maš.maš) in colophons. At the same time, Kiṣir-Assur was essentially a scholar who collected a wide range of tablets on healing arts, including medical texts which contained recipes without incantations, but we have no reason to assume that Kiṣir-Assur practiced as anything other than what he claimed to be – an exorcist.

Judging by these examples of famous scholars, we can see that Babylonian scholarship divided into various disciplines and even sub-disciplines. One area of specialization was divination and astronomy, which demanded an extensive knowledge of all kinds of omen texts, but not necessarily expertise in magic, incantations, or medicine. The other area of specialization was that of the exorcist, who needed to know a great deal about the large repertoire of Sumerian and Akkadian incantations but at the same time something about omens and medicine in general.

For centuries the learned exorcist shared his clients with another healing technician, the *asû*-"physician," who at that time was responsible for drugs and drafted and prepared prescriptions. The colophons of tablets from the Nineveh library clearly show the division between the two professions, the exorcist and physician. Medical colophons, for instance, refer to the patronage of healing gods Ninurta and Gula, while incantations almost always rely upon the assistance of gods Marduk and Ea. By the late first millennium BC, as we have seen, this distinction between exorcist and physician was breaking down.[157]

In Babylonian terms, is there any equivalent to the Greek philosopher "healing the soul"? Although not exactly a philosopher, the Babylonian exorcist had to comprehend all aspects of the cosmos and man's relationships within it. The exorcist was responsible for helping the patient to divert the anger of the petulant gods or the unseen dangers of demons, ghosts, witchcraft, black magic, or slander – in other words, treating the patient's psyche. Greek *Heilkunde*, like its Babylonian neighbor, also never freed itself from belief in magic and demons and divine intervention. In both systems, there is a recognizable component of healing the psyche (or the soul) through means other than what we call "medicine" (i.e. the use of drugs, diet, or surgery). So although the Babylonian exorcist was never a philosopher per se, by the seventh century BC he had become a scholar of the healing arts and a master of all aspects of his discipline.

Innovation

But things change, and sometimes we can even tell when they change. At some point early in the fifth century BC certain innovations were introduced into traditional Babylonian medicine. One such innovation was astral medicine, in which appropriate apotropaic and healing rituals were to be performed during propitious times determined by the zodiac. Texts describing the correspondences between rituals and zodiac signs date from the Hellenistic period, but an earlier version, dating from 619 BC, gives the same rituals without any reference to zodiac signs (Reiner 1995: 108ff.; 111). Astral medicine and astral magic were thus incorporated into traditional literature some time after this date.

Another innovation was probably introduced by a family of scribes from Uruk in Babylonia which flourished in the reign of Darius, roughly contemporary with Hippocrates himself. Anu-ikṣur was a member of this distinguished family of scholars consisting of priests and exorcists, whose work we will discuss in a later chapter. Many tablets from the family archive belong to his brother Rīmūt-Anu and his father, Šamaš-iddin, also distinguished scribes in their own right, who were active during the Persian period, c. 400 BC (Hunger 1976: No. 11; Robson 2008: 227–62). Rīmūt-Anu owned several medical tablets, each of which is significant in its own right. The first of these tablets is the so-called exorcism manual ascribed to Esagil-kīn-apli (mentioned above), which is known from copies from Assur and Nineveh in Assyrian script, as well as later copies in Babylonian script from Babylon and Sippar (Jean 2006: 63); Rīmūt-Anu's copy indicates that this important catalogue of incantation and medical texts was also studied in Uruk during the Persian period. Two other tablets in Rīmūt-Anu's possession are unique and perhaps even more important. The first of these is a list of diseases ascribed to one of four internal organs, the heart, the stomach, the lungs, and the kidneys (see Heeßel 2004: 113). Here is an extract from the final section (Hunger 1976: No. 43, 25–31):

from the kidneys	"stricture"
ditto	impotence
ditto	anal disease
ditto	muscle disease
ditto	barrenness
ditto	womb which is twisted
ditto	"gas" retention

There is no ancient explanatory commentary on this puzzling text, which appears to be a radical departure from any previous attempt at disease taxonomy within Babylonian medicine. One possibility is that each of these diseases is thought to have a "seat" or residence within a particular internal organ, which may have parallels within Hippocratic medicine (Geller 2004a: 37). In any case, external symptoms are presented as manifestations of diseases associated with internal organs, without reference to divine intervention, anger, or demonic attack. Another of Rīmūt-Anu's medical tablets is a listing of diseases according to each one's individual "nature" or "property" (*šiknu*), associating characteristic symptoms with a disease name.[158] The final section of the tablet lists ailments with the conventional designation of "Hand of a God" (e.g. "Hand of Gula," "Hand of Marduk," "Hand of Šamaš"), but redefines these terms with specific disease names, such as various skin ailments or jaundice or sores (Heeßel 2000: No. 33). As Heeßel comments on this text, "this shift of focus from the interest in the divine origin of sickness to the mechanisms of nature and the bodily origin of diseases represents, then, a small 'revolution of wisdom' within late Babylonian medicine" (Heeßel 2004: 114).

Although Rīmūt-Anu and his brother Anu-ikṣur refer to themselves by the title of "exorcists" (maš.maš), most of the medical tablets found at fifth-century Uruk typically belong to them (Hunger 1976: No. 12; Pedersén 1998: 212). Anu-ikṣur also owned the largest known collection of commentaries on medical tablets, which may not be coincidental but reflects fresh thinking about medicine and anatomy, rather than merely copying traditional medical recipes. At the same time, by the Persian period, Uruk exorcists had become the most prominent scholars of their day. A contemporary library from Uruk's Eanna temple contains some 250 tablets dealing with incantations, medicine prayers, omens, and astronomy, and the few surviving colophons on these tablets ascribe them to exorcists (maš.maš).[159] This suggests that an exorcist, in order to perform his duties properly, had to be a good all-rounder.

The mystery, in fact, is what happened to the archives of the physician, who disappeared from colophons from the Achaemenid period onward. It is possible that a late private medical archive simply remains to be found by archaeologists, but circumstantial evidence allows for other inferences to be drawn. We have many hundreds of school texts from Babylon and Sippar from the latter half of the first millennium and even a few from the first century AD. These extract tablets give students the opportunity to practice reading (or copying) a variety of texts on a single tablet, usually consisting of lexical texts, *belles lettres*, omens, personal names, and other genres; many contain extracts from incantations (see Gesche 2001: 214), but not a single extract tablet cites prescriptions or medical texts.

These late extract tablets from Babylon and Sippar, however, do not tell the whole story. Ironically, the medics seem to have disappeared from view but the medical tablets continued to be copied and used. As noted above, Irving Finkel published an archive of late Achaemenid copies of incantation and medical texts in both portrait and landscape formats; the texts are cursive and hardly look like finished library copy (Finkel 2000). Despite the fact that the tablets are more medical than magical, this archive is likely to belong to an exorcist. Another collection of such tablets belonged to a scholar named Tanittu-Bēl from Babylon, some of whose tablets can be dated to the thirteenth year of Alexander the Great, bringing us down to 323 BC (Finkel 1991).[160] Although never referring to him specifically by title, Tanittu-Bēl's archive mostly consists of incantations and related literature, including rituals for massage and fumigation. A further late archive from Uruk includes many similar tablets, copied by a versatile local exorcist named Iqīšâ, who also had an abiding interest in medicine, as we will see below.[161] The consistent picture is that despite the presence of substantial late archives belonging to diviners and exorcists, not a single contemporary medical archive is known that belonged to an *asû*-physician, either anonymously or by name.

Let us summarize our argument thus far. The system of Babylonian medicine down to the eighth century BC (prior to Hippocrates) involved collaboration between the exorcist and physician, with a clear division of textual content between incantations and medical recipes. The exorcist's training began to evolve as he familiarized himself with therapeutic remedies, as well as with the numerous genres of incantations and magical rituals.

Subtle changes occurred during the Persian period, perhaps influenced by the *Zeitgeist*; scribes and scholars began to enumerate diseases without attributing their causes to either gods or demons. It is during this same period that the *asû*-physician virtually disappears from colophons and texts, although medical texts continue to be copied and owned by scribes who are exorcists. It seems that exorcists not only incorporated medicine more fully into their curriculum, but indulged in some new thinking about medicine. But while all this was happening, where was the *asû*-physician?

Could exorcists have actually usurped the role of the physician? Herodotus famously observed that Babylonians did not have doctors, but when ill one simply lay down in the street and waited for people to come

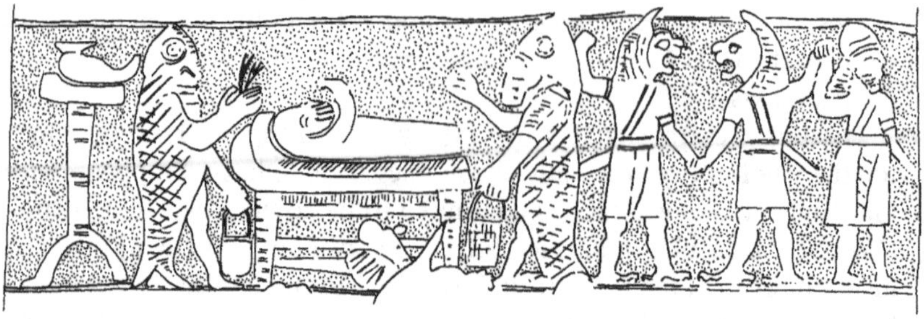

Figure 5.1 Patient being healed (Wiggermann 2007: 107, No. 1; drawing courtesy F. A. M. Wiggermann)

along and give medical advice. One wonders how Herodotus got it so wrong, since we have so much evidence about medicine in Babylonia. Perhaps Herodotus entered a temple and asked the priests about doctors, and was simply told, "we don't have any," referring to the *asû*. Herodotus then drew his own conclusions.

Whatever information or misinformation Herodotus reports, it is probably no coincidence that significant changes occurred in Babylonia in his day. We know from a famous but apocryphal legend that Hippocrates declined to take up a lucrative position as physician at Darius's court. While Hippocrates was imposing a new understanding on Greek medicine by de-emphasizing gods and demons as causes of disease, a similar *esprit* may have been taking place at the same time in Babylonia, especially among scribes from the cities of Babylon and Uruk. Babylonian scholars in the early fifth century BC not only developed a keen interest in expounding medical texts, but attempted to classify diseases without reference to deities, in more natural rather than supernatural terms. Hippocrates would probably have approved.

Ascendance of the Exorcist and Decline of the Physician

The records from colophons of tablets show that the exorcist became a dominant member of the temple elites, while other scholars, particularly *bārû* and *asû*, seem to disappear from our records. We can account for this change from various possible perspectives. The archives that we have in late periods are often from temples, which means that those professions allied to the priesthood will naturally be better represented than secular or non-priestly professions, such as the *asû*. On the other hand, there is another way of thinking about the changes that took place between the status of the two healing professionals.

By 539 BC, Cyrus the Great had conquered Babylonia, setting in motion the expansion of the Persian Empire which would eventually extend "from India to Ethiopia," as claimed in the Book of Esther. Persian rule dominated the entire Near East for the next two centuries, ushering in a period of unprecedented globalization, in which the region was united by political stability and a common language, Aramaic. Although Akkadian continued to be used as both administrative and literary language throughout Mesopotamia, Aramaic eventually replaced Akkadian as lingua franca and became the language of cross-border communication, as well as being a widely spoken language in the region. Persian influence also spread throughout the region, and certain fundamentally Persian notions of eschatology, dualism (good and evil, light and dark), and of a final epoch became widely acknowledged.

Although indigenous records are virtually non-existent, Greeks living at the Persian court have important things to say about the role of physicians and exorcists under Persian rule. Ctesias, a Greek physician and historian, claims to have been invited to serve as personal physician to Artaxerxes II (Briant 2002: 264f.). Other Greek physicians were known at the Persian court, mostly by name only, although Ctesias tells the lurid tale of one Apollinides at the court of Artaxerxes I, who fell in love with the king's sister and was buried alive after her death. Herodotus also speaks of one successful Greek physician, Democedes (Briant 2002: 265), who persuaded Darius not to execute his many Egyptian court physicians, because of their incompetence. With Greek and Egyptian doctors being prominent at the Persian court, why is there no mention of local doctors? However, these court physicians were not the only medical practitioners who served the Persian kings. Xenophon and Strabo report that Cyrus ordered medicinal plants to be collected to maintain the health of his soldiers, and Briant infers that "there is little doubt that the specialists to whom Cyrus appealed were none other than the magi" (Briant 2002: 267).

But who were these magi? Descriptions of their functions are general and vague, based mostly on eyewitness accounts by foreigners (Greeks) rather than Persian sources. Strabo describes Persian sacrifices in the simplest of terms, essentially consisting of dry wood being burned on an altar, often with aromatic substances being added and incantations being recited by magi. This type of offering most closely resembles Babylonian fumigation rituals, used in both magic and medicine. Essentially all we know from Greek eyewitness accounts is that magi worshipped at fire altars, which is hardly remarkable, nor do we have any idea of the special expertise or training required to perform such ritual tasks. The Greek term *magoi* also had pejorative connotations, as in the Hippocratic corpus (*On the Sacred Disease* 1 2), which refers to *magoi* along with quacks and charlatans (see Burkert 2004: 108–9).

The main deities worshipped were Ahura-Mazda and the sun (Mithra), and a goddess Anahita, whose character was influenced by Mesopotamian Ištar (Briant 2002: 245–54). The most distinctive feature of Persian ritual was the sacrifice of horses to gods, which is unprecedented in Mesopotamia. Although actual Persian sources on the activities of the magi are relatively scarce, the main sacerdotal activities of the magi are clear, and we know that they relied upon blood sacrifices and incantations for their rituals. According to one classical author, Diogenes Laertius, the magi insisted that only their prayers and incantations were heard by the gods, and for this reason the magi practiced divination as well; other sources speak of magi acting against demons (Burkert 2004: 120f.). The sketchy descriptions of the interests of the magi are actually quite close to the activities of the exorcist in Babylonia, whose chief function, as described by Paul-Alain Beaulieu, was "to prevent and conjure up the punishments sent by the gods" (Beaulieu 2007: 479). There are a few references to the *magušu* in Akkadian, referring to the activities of the magus as a Persian official/priest who had considerable power within the temple administration.[162] The word *magušu* soon falls out of use in Akkadian, possibly because the role of the magus was so closely identified with that of the *mašmaššu* that the loanword became redundant.

Magi were prominent at the Persian court, and there is little to distinguish them from Babylonian priests who performed similar functions. The *mašmaššu* would certainly qualify as the Babylonian priests corresponding most closely to magi. Although Persian policy under Cyrus and his successors intended to avoid suppressing local religion in favor of Persian religious practice, nevertheless the social status and prestige of the magi may have influenced Babylonian society under Persian domination.

Hence, new conditions introduced by the Persian court influenced what happened in Mesopotamia proper during this period and afterwards. First, the fact that Persian kings preferred foreign to local physicians may have had a role in reducing the prestige of Babylonian physicians, at least as far as the ruling classes were concerned. The downgrading of the local Babylonian *asû*, for some unknown reason, may partly explain why this profession all but disappears from Akkadian records. It may be that the *asû* was no longer considered to be an established profession, although non-literate classes no doubt used his services. Still, since *asûtu* was still being copied by scribes, it seems that exorcists had taken over knowledge of these texts.

Second, the prominence of magi at the Persian court may explain why the exorcist's own stock in trade rose in relation to other priests, since he becomes the dominant figure in later temple archives, judging by colophons and other data. The advanced social and professional status of the magi may have influenced the situation in Babylonia, where the expanding scholarly interests of the *mašmaššu*-clans seemed to have dominated the scene from the Persian period onwards.[163]

See also Daniel 4:4, in which Nebuchadnezzar has a dream and assembles his scholars to interpret it: *harṭumîm, ašapîm, haldîm*, and *gezarîm*. The *harṭumîm* (of whom Daniel, under his Babylonian name Belshazar, held the title *rab harṭumîm*) are dream interpreters (in this context, see Radner 2009: 224). The *ašapîm* are exorcists, from Akkadian *āšipu* (rather than *mašmaššu*, which is not loaned into Aramaic). *Haldîm* were Chaldaeans (astrologers), and *gezarîm* (lit. cutters, dissectors) are diviners. Which would correspond to magi? We would suggest *ašapîm* (*āšipu*) as the closest match, considering the involvement of magi in both magic and rituals. The Book of Daniel, as a detached witness, probably reflects with some accuracy the status of exorcists in the Neo-Babylonian court under Persian rule.

6

Medical Training: MD or PhD?

Little is known about the actual late schools, except for what can be derived from the numerous exercise tablets which have been found in excavations from sites like Babylon, Nippur, and Sippar (Gesche 2001; Lucas 1979; Cavigneaux 1981). A scribal school may have consisted of a single scholar (*ummânu*) with a small number of students (between two and four) at any one time, for a course of study which lasted some 10 years (Wiggermann 2008: 211). If this is the case, the intimate relationship between teacher and pupils could easily have fostered conditions under which the master's interpretations of texts were preserved as oral tradition by successive generations of students. These traditions, then, would have formed the basis for later commentary texts, in the form of notes on how the master understood an anonymous *textus receptus* of the scribal curriculum.

The institutional background is important if one is trying to establish whether specific training was available to scholars who acted as physicians or exorcists. Although it is a given that in the ancient and medieval world no such recognized qualifications existed, nevertheless we do find designations of various levels of scribal training in colophons of tablets, and these might provide some relevant information. A good example of the various stages of training occurs in a tablet from Assur emanating from the scribal family of *asû*-physicians under Esarhaddon, probably dating from c. 670 BC. The tablet's colophon reads:

> First extract, finished. Written by Shulgi-enu, (impressed with) the fingernail of the apprentice scribe (*šamallû*) and novice (*agašgû*), disciple (*šanduppû*) of Urad-Nanaya, "specialist in medicine,"[164] disciple (*šanduppû*) of Eṭēru, Assur scribe (*ṭupšarru*) and disciple (*šanduppû*) of Adad-uballiṭ, Assur scribe. (*JMC* 10 [2007]: 14)

Here we see several levels of scribal attainment, on a tablet which is lengthy and full of complicated medical data but nicely written. On the other hand, Shulgi-enu's tablet does contain erasures as well as many tiny glosses which translate logograms which were difficult for or unfamiliar to a student scribe (and many of which are too small to be legible today). In fact, many of these glosses represent the same kind of notes that occur in medical commentary tablets.[165] Occasionally, Shulgi-enu seems to gloss words incorrectly, or at least over-interprets text, as in one case in which the *materia medica* are to be heated over coals (l. 57) but the scribe has glossed "frit" (*nitku*, a type of glass) for coals, which seems unlikely. Some other glosses seem very elementary: the young Shulgi-enu glosses two Sumerograms which are extremely common in medical texts, meaning "you dry" and "you crush" *materia medica*.[166] In another line (41), he glosses the syllabic writing of the same word (*ta-sàk*) with *sa-ka*, since he was not sure how to read the *sàk* sign, although this is a common reading in medical texts. On the whole, we see the competent hand of an apprentice, whose writing looks professional enough but who may not have been familiar with all the particular idioms of medical literature.

These glosses may provide clues to how texts were read or rather read out in the scribal schools, at the same time as these texts were being

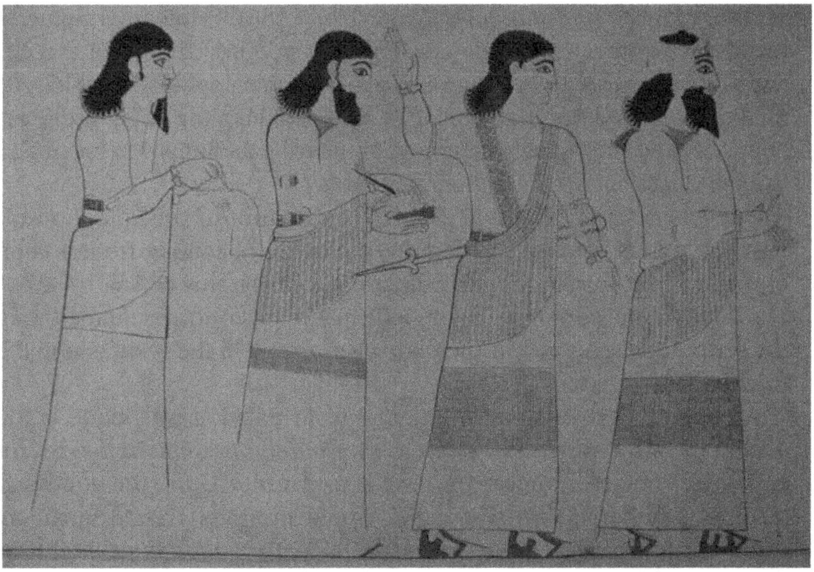

Figure 6.1 Scribes and officials from Til Barsip (ninth century BC) showing scribes writing on both leather and clay (photo Florentina Badalanova Geller)

expounded by the master scribe (*ummânu*). We would like to know whether the terms used in Shulgi-enu's colophon for "scribal apprentice" (*šamallû*), "novice" (*agašgû*), and "disciple" (*šanduppû*), imply some kind of hierarchy of recognized qualifications for a scribe who specialized in copying medical texts; even if he could copy them, does this make him a doctor? Let us look at the qualifications of other students and their status within the scribal school, judging by colophons of other tablets.

Academic Titles

The most common designations of a scribe were *ṭupšarru* "scribe" and *šamallû* "merchant, agent," and both of these terms could be modified by *ṣehru*, "junior."[167] Numerous tablets from libraries and archives are copied by scribes who refer to themselves as *ṭupšarru*, *šamallû*, or *agašgû*, and in such cases we conclude that they are "library" copies, rather than simply school exercise tablets that could be discarded. The question is whether these titles reflect some sort of progression within scribal training. An answer to this question might decide whether a physician in Babylonia in the late first millennium BC could have earned some recognized qualifications as a healer or practitioner.

For instance, the term *agašgû* "novice" can refer to either a physician (*asû*) or exorcist (*mašmaššu*) (Hunger 1968: 158).[168] In earlier Sumerian texts, this word refers to the academically poorest student in the class and not necessarily the youngest. When used in colophons of tablets, it is unlikely that a later Babylonian scribe would refer to himself as a "dunce." We can probably assume that the original Sumerian meaning of this word had changed a millennium later.

One Assur scribe, Nabû-lē'i, puts his signature to the colophon of a medical text as "novice physician" (*asû agašgû*), coming from a family of Assur scribes who were not themselves physicians (*BAM* 1 4 27).[169] The tablet in question is a list of medicinal plants or drugs, and although the script looks competent there are clear errors in the text (as noted by Köcher, *BAM* 1 p. xi).

A copy of a tablet from an original from Babylon was made by one Nabû-eṭir, who describes himself as *šamallû mašmaššu agašgû*, an apprentice novice exorcist; the text is a hymn to Gula, the goddess of healing (Lambert 1967a: 115). We would interpret this to mean that Nabû-eṭir had achieved the academic status of *šamallû* in general terms (whatever this might mean), but he also achieved the rank of *agašgû* in his work on academic exorcism, during his scholarly career.

We get some idea about the academic hierarchy in Sultantepe from tablet colophons.

1 Nabû-eṭir from Sultantepe describes himself as a "junior apprentice" (*šamallû ṣehru*) (Hunger 1968: No. 402) and "disciple" (*mar mummu*) of someone whose name is unfortunately broken. The term *mar mummi* is unusual; the *mummu* was actually a rather grandiose name for the scribal school, literally "workshop," named after the *bīt mummi* in the temple, the workshop where idols were restored. The *bīt mummi* was also a place associated with esoteric knowledge.[170]

2 A more complex Sultantepe colophon tells us that Nabû-rihtu-uṣur was, like Nabû-eṭir above, "junior apprentice" (*šamallû ṣehru*) and "disciple" (*mar mummi*) of Nabû-aha-iddin, the "head" scribe (lúsag) (Hunger 1968: No. 354 [= *STT* 38]). The "head" scribe Nabû-aha-iddin also identifies himself elsewhere as an "apprentice" (*šamallû*) (Hunger 1968: No. 359 [= *STT* 247]), probably referring to a slightly earlier stage in his academic career. It was probably as an "apprentice" that Nabû-aha-iddin had also copied tablets for the "reading" (*tāmartu*) of Qurdī-Nergal (Hunger 1968: Nos. 386, 389 [= *STT* 161, 172; see also *STT* 203]).

3 Returning to the colophon above (Hunger 1968: No. 354 [= *STT* 38]), the junior apprentice Nabu-rihtu-uṣur and disciple of the "head" scribe Nabû-aha-iddin, had written his tablet for the "reading" (*tāmartu*) of one Qurdī-Nergal. This information allows us to establish some sort of hierarchy:

"junior apprentice" (*šamallû ṣehru*)
"disciple" (*mar mummi*) of the "head" scribe
for the "reading" by Qurdī-Nergal

The disciple Nabû-rihtu-uṣur worked under Nabû-aha-iddin (as "head"); when both these scribes functioned as *šamallû*-apprentices, their tablets were copied for "reading" by Qurdī-Nergal. Was he *ummânu*? We know Qurdī-Nergal from other colophons in which he refers to himself as a "junior apprentice" (*šamallû ṣehru*) (Hunger 1968: No. 353 [= *STT* 192]), although this probably refers to an earlier period in his academic life. Moreover, another colophon (probably written by his son) bestows upon Qurdī-Nergal the august title of "priest (*šangû*) of (the gods) Zababa and Ba'u" associated with three different Assyrian cities (Arba'il, Harran, and Sultantepe itself) (Hunger 1968: No. 373 [= *STT* 64]); this may well be a later colophon. We seem to have tablets giving us information about various phases in Qurdī-Nergal's career, beginning with his student days and ending with his position as high priest, by which time he was no longer active in the scribal school, where his son was now a scholar.

We must try to determine to what "reading" (*tāmartu*) in this case precisely refers, since these colophons show that someone "reading" held a more senior position than an apprentice or even "head" scribe. Another Sultantepe scholar, Nabu-eṭiranni, composed a tablet colophon in which he specifically refers to "reading" (*tāmartu*) on behalf of several colleagues, one of whom was a priest (*sangû*), the second an *agašgû*, the third a "junior physician" (*asû ṣehru*), and the fourth a "junior apprentice" (*šamallû ṣehru*).

> For the "reading" (*ana tāmarti*) of Bēl-aha-iddin, a priest (*šangû*), ..., [for] the "reading" of [...] an *agašgû*-apprentice, for the "reading" of Rimut-ilī, junior physician (*asû ṣehru*), and for the "reading" of Zēra-ukīn, junior *šamallû*-apprentice, hastily extracted for their "reading" (*ana tāmartišunu hanṭiš nasih*). (Hunger 1968: No. 382 [= *STT* 301])[171]

This colophon is intriguing because of the institutional information it would provide if only we understood the procedures alluded to. First of all, it shows that scholarly texts could be interdisciplinary, to be read by or for students at different levels and disciplines. Second, we can assume on *a priori* grounds that a "junior" (*ṣehru*) level is less advanced than the level itself, so that a *šamallû ṣehru* would be less advanced than a *šamallû* apprentice.

Furthermore, although the title *asû* is a professional title rather than an academic one, it may be that "junior physician" (*asû ṣehru*) designates a certain academic level of training and is hence a label which belongs exclusively to an academic context, rather than as a full-fledged professional title. One exception is the title "priest" (*šangû*) occurring in this colophon, which looks like a professional title but is possibly qualified by some term (such as "junior") in the lacuna following this word.

One important scribe of the city of Assur was Kiṣir-Assur, who was a prodigious copyist of tablets and signed many with his name and titles. We see him progress from *šamallû ṣehru* to *šamallû mašmaššu*, then to *mašmaššu*, and finally to *mašmaš bīt Assur* (Hunger 1968: 19), a kind of *cursus honorum* for scribes. This progression distinguishes between titles within the scribal school system (*šamallû*) and those borne by the professional beyond the academy, namely *mašmaššu*. The *šamallû*, whether an "apprentice" or not, copies texts within an academic context, and the title is dropped once the scribe takes up a position outside the scribal school. This is the same progression we noted above in Qurdī-Nergal's career from "junior apprentice" (*šamallû ṣehru*) to priest.

The Meaning of ana tāmarti "for Reading"

There are a number of ways that a tablet could be used within academic contexts, according to the many colophons which we have. One rather uncommon expression is *ana tahsistu*, meaning the tablet is written "as an *aide-mémoire*." In other cases, the tablet could be read *ana ihzi*, for the "grasp" or understanding of the reader, or as a "norm for learning." A colophon of an astronomical tablet records that the scribe wrote the tablet *ana ahazišu*, "for his grasp," referring to his own understanding of the task (Neugebauer 1955: 117 [No. 192: 5]). A more common expression is that a tablet is written *ana šitassi*, for "reading out" of the text. The colophon provides nothing in the way of context, so we cannot tell whether "reading out" implies formal recitation or simply reading the tablet aloud (as was normal practice).

Perhaps the most intriguing expression is *ana tāmarti*, for the "reading" (lit. "viewing") of the tablet (discussed above). Occasionally words adapt to new meanings. In later periods, for instance, *tāmartu* takes on special significance, since the *bīt tāmarti* refers to the Greek theatre in Babylon, literally "house of viewing" (van der Spek 2001: 447). The expression *ana tāmarti* appears in colophons in Sultantepe (late eighth century BC), as well as in Assurbanipal's official royal colophons from Nineveh which insist that the king himself personally wrote, checked, and collated the tablets in his library, all far from likely. These colophons claim credit for Assurbanipal in the first person: "I wrote, checked, and collated this tablet from the collection of the scholars, I used it for the 'viewing' (*tāmartu*) of my majesty within my palace."[172] Considering the anonymous scribal culture of Babylonia, it is surprising to find such a claim expressed in the first person referring to the king; the expression *ana tāmartu* may simply allude to Assurbanipal's self-proclaimed literacy (Fales 2001: 43; Villard 1997: 135–49). There is no reason to give him credit beyond that.

The term *tāmartu*, however, is also used by a scholar we have already met, Nabû-zukup-kēnu, who incorporated a fair amount of personal information in his colophons (see Frahm 1999). At the end of an astronomical omen tablet, for instance, he writes: "for the *tāmarti* of my son, for half a year … I 'thickened' (i.e. worsened) my eyesight, and checked it *hastily* and collated it" (Hunger 1968: No. 299). This is a remarkable statement about monitoring his son's progress, but what is meant by *ana tāmarti*? The colophon records that "he *had it written* for his (own?) reading" (Hunger 1968: No. 297); in other words, Nabû-zukup-kēnu did not actually copy the tablet but employed it for his "reading" (*tāmartu*).

Further clues are provided by somewhat earlier Sultantepe tablets, which use this expression in a conventional way. One Sultantepe colophon comments that a scribe: "wrote (the tablet) and collated it for his (own?) reading" (*ana tāmartišu*) (*STT* 136). What do we make of this? The semantics of the verb *amāru*, to "see, view," include "read a tablet," as well as to "check" or "inspect" or even to "see the results" of a mathematical calculation.

We return to a Sultantepe tablet (*STT* 301) which we discussed above in relation to various categories of scribal "apprentices" mentioned in the colophon. The tablet was copied for "reading" by other colleagues for a specific purpose, which may have something to do with the fact that it too is a type of commentary.[173] These colleagues are not young students but already have professional qualifications; one is a priest (*sangû*), another is a "physician" (*asû*), although still part of the academy. It seems clear that the meaning of *tāmartu* is more than just reading, but has more to do with an academic scrutiny of the tablet itself. Since the two major roles of schools and school training are to teach and examine students, it is possible that *tāmartu* refers in this case to an *examination* or examining of students, inspecting or evaluating their accomplishments. This would also make sense for Nabû-zukup-kēnu's tablet for the *tāmartu* of his son's work, which he complains nearly caused him to go blind. It is hardly coincidental that this kind of academic terminology appears in colophons of commentary tablets, which represent the upper-level work of the academy.

Another unusual reference to *tāmartu* occurs in a Late Babylonian esoteric commentary tablet, which is certainly from an academic milieu. The text deals with astrology and omen matters, and its colophon categorizes it as a text coming "from the 'questions and answers' (*maš'altu*) of a 'scholar' (*ummânu*)" (Biggs 1968: 52ff.; see also Finkel 2006: 141). This genre of "questions and answers" is known from Greek and Latin apocrypha as a type of hermeneutics, as well as from medieval and later apocryphal literature, and refers to a special category of erotapocritic literature, usually referring to esoteric subjects.[174] These tablets are all said to have originated as "questions and answers" (*maš'altu*) of an *ummânu*-scholar.

One esoteric commentary which refers to itself as a *maš'altu* ("questions and answers") is a single-column tablet belonging to Nabû-šum-lišir, from a priestly family devoted to the god Bēl-ṣarbi. The colophon then says that "a lamentation priest (*kalû*) of (the god) Bēl-ṣarbi wrote and checked the tablet for his *tāmartu*" (Biggs 1968: 54, 21). The question is why a lamentation priest, who functioned as a temple singer, would be interested in a tablet dealing with astrology and omens; the tablet itself is hardly intelligible to anyone not immersed in esoteric scholarship, associating astrology with unnatural or unusual births which were seen as portentous. Whatever the reason, the word *tāmartu* here means more than merely perusal of the tablet, and in fact must have a more definitive purpose. We may presume that the *tāmartu* has some specific academic role, similar to other cases discussed above. We suggest that this tablet represents an *examination* of the lamentation priest, to demonstrate his scholarly credentials. The person doing the examining (i.e. *tāmartu*) is the most senior authority in the academy, which is reflected in the hierarchical statements of various academic colophons.

Finally, the term *tāmartu* appears in the opening line of the standard list of exorcism incipits ascribed to the twelfth-century BC scholar Esagil-kīn-apli (Jean 2006: 63ff. [= *KAR* 44]): "Incipits of the Series belonging to the art of exorcism (*mašmaššūtu*), established (*kunnu*) for instruction (*ihzu*) and testing (*tāmartu*), all to be read out." The terms here are relevant to an academic context, since the line informs us that various editions of incantations have been compiled and "fixed" (*kunnu*) for academic "instruction" (*ihzu*) as well as for "testing" (*tāmartu*). No other meaning of *tāmartu* quite fits this context, since "reading" or "viewing" text editions of incantations would hardly follow "instruction." This important incipit refers specifically to the two main tasks of a scribal school, as mentioned above: teaching and examining pupils.

The Case of Anu-ikṣur of Uruk

An archive of medical and medically related commentary tablets from Uruk, from the fifth century BC, belonging to an exorcist named Anu-ikṣur, has a lot to tell us generally about procedures within the ancient scribal academies. In my view, Anu-ikṣur was more than a mere copyist of tablets or even collector of tablets, since it is most likely that he was the actual master who was responsible for many of the Uruk commentaries from this period. No less than 11 commentary tablets were labeled as coming from "the mouth of the 'professor' (*ummânu*), the lecture (*malsût*) of Anu-ikṣur" (see Hunger 1976: No. 50, 42; Robson 2008: 233–5). Could Anu-ikṣur have been the *ummânu*-"professor" mentioned in the colophons, whose oral teachings were being committed to writing?

One argument in favor of Anu-ikṣur being the author of these commentaries rests upon the meaning of the phrase, *ana malsûti*, "for the lecture of." The use of the term *malsûtu* "lecture" is not prevalent outside of Uruk. There is the exception of several appearances of the term in the colophons of several medical texts copied by an important Assur scribe, Kiṣit-Nabû, but all of these Assur tablets were copied from Uruk originals (*BAM* 52, 106, 147). This scribe, probably a contemporary of Assurbanipal, was an exorcist from an important family of exorcists (Pedersén 1986: 46), who signed his colophons with the notation, *ana tāmartišu* "for his reading" (i.e. for examination purposes) or in one case, *ana malsutišu*, "for his lecture."[175] The term *malsûtu* appears in Assur in a copy of a normal medical tablet, while the term *malsûtu*, as used later in Uruk by Anu-ikṣur, refers exclusively to commentary tablets.[176]

One possibility is that, if Anu-ikṣur himself was *ummânu*, any tablet designated as being from the "mouth of the *ummânu*" could have been composed by his students who took notes, much in the same way that Aristotle's students provided posterity with his thinking on natural science. Supporting evidence for this idea exists, since several Uruk colophons specify that although the tablet belonged to Anu-ikṣur, it was his son Anu-ušallim who actually copied the tablet (Robson 2008: 235f.), which we would understand as transcribing and recording Anu-ikṣur's lecture notes. The same pattern occurs in later Uruk colophons, in the tablets of the Uruk scholar Šamaš-eṭir, copied by Anu-aba-utēr, who later becomes an *ummânu* in his own right. Anu-aba-utēr's own tablets are copied, some dozen years later, by younger scribes, including his own nephew (Robson 2008: 248–51). The pattern appears to be that if commentary tablets are said to come "from the mouth of the *ummânu*," the owner of the tablet is the *ummânu*, but if colophons omit this expression but refer by name to the tablet owner, he is the *ummânu* and the tablet has been copied by a son or disciple. Tablets ascribed to Anu-ikṣur follow both of these patterns.

Anu-ikṣur's title of "junior exorcist" (*mašmaššu ṣehru*) (Hunger 1976: No. 41, 11′) places him firmly within the academy,[177] although we should ask whether this status rendered him sufficiently qualified to be considered an *ummânu*. Could one be an *ummânu* and *mašmaššu ṣehru* at the same time? One thing is clear, that the title of *ummânu* is never actually conveyed in colophons on the writer or owner of the tablet, nor does this title ever seem to be one of the hierarchical levels in scribal schools.[178] In other words, Anu-ikṣur is never referred to as *ummânu* in colophons, nor are any other scribes granted this title, nor do we see the status of *ummânu* as part of the career structure of scribal schools, as one might have expected. One does not seem to progress from "apprentice" to "professor" in any professional hierarchy.

This means that the expression "from the mouth of the *ummânu*" (*ša pî ummâni*) simply means, "on expert authority." For the moment, therefore, our hypothesis is that Anu-ikṣur was responsible for composing these commentaries, that it is his name which gives the commentaries authority, and that these notes belong to his lectures in the scribal academy.[179] On the other hand, it may be that everyone simply knew who the *ummânu* at any time was within the school, without having to mention him by name, in the same way that the title "Pope" is sufficient in itself to identify the person holding this position.

Another supporting argument for the "owner" of a commentary tablet being its "author" is this: commentary tablets do not usually duplicate each other in the way that other texts are duplicates. Commentary texts did not operate within the curriculum in the same way as the literature upon which they were commenting. Even in cases in which several medical commentaries were composed in different scribal schools on the same original composition, the commentaries differ from each other. A good example is provided by three commentaries expounding the first tablet of the Diagnostic Handbook. All three commentaries are from Uruk (with one belonging to Anu-ikṣur) and are said to have originated as "questions and answers" (*maš'altu*) of an *ummânu*.[180] Three extant commentaries on the same text do *not* duplicate each other. The fact that we have three commentaries on the opening tablet of the Diagnostic Handbook shows not only how popular it was, but also how difficult it was to understand. The fact that commentaries are not duplicated shows that we are dealing here with an innovative literary genre of the first millennium.[181]

Colophons of cuneiform tablets frequently mention the copyist or owner of a tablet but rarely refer to the person who actually composed a literary or scientific text. There are a few exceptions. A small number of texts are ascribed to specific authors, such as Sīn-leqe-unnini, who is credited with being the author of Gilgamesh, and Kabti-ilāni-Marduk, who composed the Erra Epic, while the authors of the Poem of the Righteous Sufferer (*Ludlul bel nēmeqi*) and a Hymn to Gula are both known by name (Foster 2007: 6). Scientific literature in particular is characteristically anonymous, with libraries of tablets being copied generation after generation by local scribes with no indication of authorship. Nevertheless, three Babylonian scholars, Šuma-iddina (Greek Soudinos), Kidinnu, and Nabû-rimanni, who appear in colophons of Babylonian astronomical tablets, were known to Strabo *by name* (as well as to other Greek authors), implying that these late scholars were either great authors or great teachers

(Schnabel 1923: 222–7; Neugebauer 1955: 1 16). It is hard to imagine that mere scribes as copyists would have made enough of an impact to become known internationally, and we must assume that these Babylonian scholars were, in fact, interpreters and teachers of Babylonian science.

Returning to Uruk colophons, our supposition is that the Uruk scholar Anu-ikṣur, when referring to his lectures, means just that: he is the one who composed the commentary for use in his lecture, which would be the basis for expounding the difficult terminology of the basic text, e.g. from the Diagnostic Handbook or a medical text; Anu-ikṣur might also provide a phrase from which a discussion of medical principles could take place. The fact that anonymity in Babylonian scientific writing is beginning to change, from the Persian domination onwards (after 525 BC), is in keeping with what we know from Greek writing from the same period, when authors began writing treatises in their own name.

While it is difficult to decide the question of scribal qualifications based upon internal evidence only, a brief glance at what was happening in the Greco-Roman world provides additional perspective on this question. The best evidence for an ancient medical curriculum comes from third-century BC Alexandria, where we find discussion of what subjects were appropriate for the study of medicine. The medical curriculum of that important centre of learning included medical lexicography and critical literary analyses of medical texts, especially in reference to the Hippocratic corpus, which were by then difficult to comprehend (Valance 2000: 101). This is not so different from Uruk commentaries.

Within the Greco-Roman scene in general, rhetoric and philosophy remained core disciplines of higher education, and these subjects were applied to medicine as well. Rhetoric was essential for a learned doctor to counter competition from others who might be providing health services, especially if practitioners of folk remedies were themselves illiterate. Persuasive rhetoric combined with a grounding in philosophy and logic would put the doctor ahead of his competitors, since Greco-Roman medicine was essentially an entrepreneurial affair (Valance 2000: 98f.).

There is no evidence from Babylonian schools that rhetoric was part of the curriculum, but the varied nature of training in Alexandria may reflect changes in curriculum in Babylonia. Instead of intense specialization based on professional training, the Late Babylonian scribal curriculum may have become more comprehensive, with a student-exorcist being expected to have a more well-rounded general exposure to many genres of texts, including medicine and divination. This might partly explain why so many different genres of tablets were being copied by exorcists or students of exorcism, as can be seen in late archives such as at Uruk.

7

Uruk Medical Commentaries

We need to explore whether ancient medical commentaries may provide clues to contemporary Babylonian medical theory or offer more general medical aphorisms which help interpret Babylonian medical texts. What we are specifically looking for are statements in medical commentaries which are somewhat more complex than the typical A = B word definitions, or deconstructing Sumerian terms (logograms) by etymologizing component parts, often incorrectly. It is the commentaries which most likely reflect the actual teachings of the *ummânu*.[182] We can neither entertain or rule out (without supporting evidence) the possibility of formal discourses, since colophons speak of texts being hastily extracted for a "lecture" (*malsûtu*), but one can only surmise what this term actually means, in institutional terms. Nevertheless, medical commentaries offer opportunities for trying to reconstruct, at least for the latest periods of Babylonian medicine, some kind of theory of medicine recorded by Babylonian scholars themselves.

Commentaries on the Diagnostic Handbook and General Themes of Prognosis

Among the most important and longest ancient commentary tablets are three commentaries from Uruk, expounding the first tablet of the Diagnostic Handbook, referred to above (George 1991); all probably date from the fifth century BC. One commentary was written by Enlil-bēlšunu, an academic (i.e. "junior") exorcist (*mašmaššu ṣehru*).[183] A second commentary was signed by Anu-ikṣur, probably a contemporary of Enlil-bēlšunu (George 1991: 152, 162). A third Uruk commentary looks very much like the hand of Anu-ikṣur as well, although the colophon is broken. Would the same scholar have put his stylus to two different commentaries on the same text? It is certainly possible that Anu-ikṣur was responsible for both Uruk commentaries on the same text.[184]

The first two tablets of the Diagnostic Handbook are extraordinary and differ markedly from the rest of the series. These tablets are concerned with general omens, similar to terrestrial omens, while the rest of the composition is mostly concerned with prognosis and diagnosis (see Fincke 2006–7: 146). Specifically, the omens of the first tablets of the Diagnostic Handbook deal with signs and portents which the exorcist encounters *en route* to the patient's house, and these signs are open to divinatory and lexical interpretation, i.e. they are a means to determine whether the patient will live or die. This type of omen was probably, at least in its original form, more the province of the *bārû*-diviner than the exorcist. It may therefore be the case that these commentaries were required in order to make the opening tablets of the Diagnostic Handbook more relevant to medicine. There are some general medical principles expressed within these commentaries, which should be noted.

Pandemic fever

The first tablet of the Diagnostic Handbook records an omen stipulating that if the exorcist, while going to the patient, happens to spot a black, white, or red pig, various deductions can be made regarding the likely fate of the patient:

> If he (the exorcist) sees a black pig: that patient may die; (alternatively) he may suffer acutely but then recover.
> If he (the exorcist) sees a white pig: that patient may get better; (alternatively) stress (*dannatu*) may take hold of him.
> If he (the exorcist) sees a red pig: that patient may die within three months, (alternatively) within three days.
> If he (the exorcist) sees a spotted pig: that patient may die from dropsy; it is worrying, one should not approach him. (*TDP* 1 6–9; George 1991: 142f.)

The Diagnostic Handbook makes several general medical observations about the patient which reoccur elsewhere in diagnostic omens: the illness may be fatal, or alternatively prolonged and curable; the illness may improve but the patient will still suffer considerable distress; the patient may survive for a determined period, or the illness may be beyond hope and perhaps contagious (not to be approached). All of these medical predictions are taken up in the commentaries, which try to make medical sense of this passage. First of all, both Enlil-bēlšunu and Anu-ikṣur agree that the Sumerian logogram used for "pig" (šah) can also indicate *li'bu*-fever, as is known from an ancient lexicon (see George 1991: 146f., 155). In other words, the word for "pig" might be a secret coding for a common illness (pandemic?) rather than simply an ominous sign, and the exorcist is looking for an indication as to whether the illness might be fatal or whether the patient will eventually survive after a protracted period. We will see how this idea plays out in the commentaries.

Fasting

Both scholars add a qualifying statement (although not in the same sequence) about a medical prediction that the patient "may get better; (alternatively) stress (*dannatu*) may take hold of him." The commentators reinterpret the meaning of Akkadian *dannatu*, based upon another common meaning for *dannatu* as "famine": "if the patient has experienced *malnourishment* (*dannatu*) he may get better, if he has not experienced *malnourishment* (*dannatu*), he may die" (George 1991: 146 6a–b).[185] Elsewhere in the Diagnostic Handbook, an infant (or young child) faces a fatal prognosis because its stomach cannot retain food and its teeth fall out, and it will experience "malnourishment" (*dannatu*) for 15–20 days. Similarly in the Diagnostic Handbook, a patient may die if lack of nourishment (*dannatu*) has taken hold of him, to the extent that he has reduced his intake of food, his lung whistles, and he has fever (Heeßel 2000: 257: 71 [= Labat 1951: 22]). The Enlil-bēlšunu and Anu-ikṣur commentaries both rely upon a general rule, that *if a patient fasted, he may recover; if not, he was likely to die*, applied in this specific case to *li'bu*-fever, which was the agreed interpretation of "pig" in this context. Similar points were often raised in Greek medicine, such as the Hippocratic aphorism stating that "diseases caused by over-eating are cured by fasting; those caused by starvation are cured by feeding up" (Lloyd 1983: 266).[186]

Contagion

The last omen given in the extract above stated that seeing a spotted pig can indicate dropsy (*aganutillû*),[187] and if the patient's condition becomes worrying (*naqud*), one should not approach the patient (*TDP* 1 9). This statement encounters no comment from either scholar, perhaps because no medical logic can be found to support this omen. However, the rule not to approach a patient with an acute illness is applied by Anu-ikṣur to another diagnostic omen: "If an ox butts him, that patient is in worrying state, one should not approach him" (*TDP* 1 18). The commentary relies upon an alternative designation of the Sumerian logogram for "ox" (gu_4) as "ghost" (gedim), which makes the rule more generally applicable and medically relevant; seeing a ghost (threatening disease) suggests the danger of contagion, to be avoided by not approaching the patient (George 1991: 148 18b).

Quarantine

Both Enlil-bēlšunu and Anu-ikṣur rely on the image of the "black pig" to introduce a method of hermeneutics which involves citing relevant explanatory literature. Both scholars deduce a passage from terrestrial omens (Šumma ālu) to explain the idea of an exorcist seeing a black pig; the omen states that "if a pig enters a bedroom, a captive woman (*asirtu*) will enter the owner's house";[188] Anu-ikṣur adds the comment that "the expression 'captive women' (*asirtu*) actually means to confine (*esēr*) the patient" (George 1991: 146 6b), perhaps referring to quarantine (Akk. *esertu/isirtu*), and hence a medical "rule" is once again being promulgated.[189]

In effect, the commentaries of Enlil-bēlšunu and Anu-ikṣur add important medical information to a text from the Diagnostic Handbook, which itself looks like a casuistic omen. Once the commentators agree that the exorcist sighting a "black pig" may in fact refer to seeing *li'bu*-fever, the subject changes from divination to medicine. Both scholars relate this equation[190] to another omen, also referring to unusual behavior of a pig, but now reinterpreting the omen. Instead of a "concubine" entering the house (causing domestic strife), "confinement" (a homonym) befalls the house, which was a way of protecting against a type of fever occasionally described as a pandemic.[191]

Rule of thumb

Anu-ikṣur took an interest in the Diagnostic Handbook observation that "the patient may die within three months or within three days" (*TDP* 1 8), which is vague and requires clarifying. Anu-ikṣur's comment gives the needed clarification: "If the patient is in a worrying state (*naqud*), he can die within three days; if he is not in a worrying state, he can die within three months" (George 1991: 148 8b–c). The time phase of prognosis is related to the perceived severity of the illness, and this statement intends to provide a general guideline for prognosis upon which the practitioner can rely.

Anatomy

The Uruk archives record other commentaries on the Diagnostic Handbook which are not found in other libraries, probably produced by Anu-ikṣur for his students. One Uruk tablet (Hunger 1976: No. 40) is a short commentary on the Diagnostic Handbook Tablet 36 and although the underlying Diagnostic Handbook text is broken, we can partially reconstruct the text from the commentary itself. The source text refers to aspects of hair on the head and prognoses which can be derived from the state of the scalp. This particular passage refers to a *harimtu*, a prostitute, who is "swollen and belches; she will die." The obvious question is why? The commentary explains as the reason for her symptoms that she has been struck on the head, with a clarifying explanation that "being hit on the head is being struck on the brain."[192] There next follows an unidentified quotation, "thus did I recite a lament for you," but the relevance is unclear; perhaps the idea is that an incantation or lament should be recited at this stage, because the situation is hopeless. The commentary returns to the subject of scalp hair, which is why it is appended to this particular section of the Diagnostic Handbook. "The hair on her head is red" (presumably because of the blood) appears to be the actual diagnostic omen, and a commentary then explains that "red" can be interpreted as "strewn" (or "thin on top"), which may allude to baldness or alopecia. The association of ideas is that one case of hair being red when caused by flowing blood is related to a second case when the natural hair colour is red.

The next symptom quoted in this same commentary refers to the eyes, stating that "the 'vine' of the patient's eyes is stretched so that the eyeball pops out,"[193] and this same comment occurs verbatim in another commentary on the Diagnostic Handbook in which bloodshot eyes immediately follow upon symptoms of baldness.[194] No other connection between these two commentaries can be established, and statements like these may simply represent anatomical lore which was widely circulating at the time.

The commentary turns next to the nose: "At its base is dripping[195] (which makes it) difficult to arouse (someone) or put (one to sleep)." The commentary explains this as "sneezing,[196] the nature[197] of which does not change." These last two comments appear to be simple medical observations.

Causes

Still looking for general principles among Uruk commentaries, we find a commentary on Tablet 3 of the Diagnostic Handbook:

> If a man is hot from his head to his midriff, but cold from his midriff to his feet, a murderous god has affected him; he has stolen *something secret*[198] from a ship and god of the harbour "seized" him, he will malinger but get better. (Labat 1951: 28, 86–7)

The commentary adds, "whatever (it was) of the boat which he stole, [*he returned*]" (Hunger 1976: No. 29, 4′); the restoration is conjectural but plausibly explains how a man could be seized by a deity/demon on moral grounds but still escape death by an act of contrition, which the original text fails to explain. The commentary, in this case, makes the traditional text more "rational" by explaining how death was avoided.[199]

The same passage of the Diagnostic Handbook reads, "if he is ill from head to midriff but is healthy from his midriff to his feet, he will be ill by the new moon; his illness will be prolonged but he will get better" (Labat 1951: 28, 89). The commentary adds one comment, "the outgoing month" (Hunger 1976: No. 29, 6′), meaning that the illness which already began in the previous month will persist at least until the next month. Vagueness is clarified in the commentary.

As we have seen, commentaries often function by comparing different texts, or by quoting from another text as a way of bringing traditional or relevant material to bear on a particular subject. One of the Uruk medical commentaries, probably belonging to Anu-ikṣur, expounds the following line of the Diagnostic Handbook, Tablet 4: "if a man's temple is affected (lit. struck), Hand of the Sibitti."[200] The symptom expressed here is so general and uninformative that the text itself tells us little of value in medical or diagnostic terms.

To explain this line further, Anu-ikṣur quotes from the first tablet of the Erra Epic, a relatively late composition (c. 700 BC) which deals with plague and death as one of its main themes. The commentary quotes the following line from the epic: "Anu, king of the gods, had sex with (Mother) Earth, she bore him seven gods and they were named the Divine Seven (*Sibitti*)" (Erra I 29; see Hunger 1976: No. 30, 16–17). Anu-ikṣur's remark is intended to explain the disease name "Hand of the Sibitti"; the Sibitti are a group of seven gods who also qualify as demons and are hence responsible for disease and misfortune, well attested in incantations.

Is there anything other than literary allusion to this quote from the Erra Epic? The point being made is that the seven Sibitti gods or demons are no less significant than Šamaš, Ištar, or other gods mentioned in this same context, but the Sibitti have an ancient pedigree going back to creation itself. The commentary asserts that although we recognize the label "Hand of a God" as a general label for disease (Heeßel 2000:

356f.), in fact the cosmological associations behind disease names need to be taken into consideration and may offer relevant background information.

The question is whether the reference in the Erra passage to the Sibitti being spawned by Anu (heaven) and Mother Earth may actually have some bearing on the diagnosis. The commentary itself provides the excuse for posing this question, since it interprets the part of the body concerned in a strange fashion. The logogram for the temple of the head is sag.ki, which Anu-ikṣur deconstructs (in good commentary fashion): SAG = man, KI = woman (Hunger 1976: No. 30, 15). These equations, while unexpected and surprising, surely have some bearing on the diagnosis, but it is not yet clear what the connection is until we look further into the commentary itself.

The source text from the Diagnostic Handbook Tablet 4 records two other symptoms of the temple which read, "If the temple on the right/left hurts him and his right/left eye is inflamed and he sheds tears," it is the "Hand of the Ghost" (alternatively "Hand of Ištar") (Labat 1951: 36, 31–2). Anu-ikṣur then takes up the meaning of "shedding (tears)": "pouring out (tears) refers to a man's wife" (Hunger 1976: No. 30, 14). The point of the passage now acquires quite a different meaning: the symptoms affecting the temple are concerned with *psychological* rather than *physical* symptoms, since the commentary suggests that tears flow because of a trauma associated with a man's wife (either the patient's own wife or someone else's). When all comments on this passage are assembled, a new picture emerges: health problems of the "temple" (usually associated with migraine) may relate to sexual relations, and symptoms of depression (shedding tears) may result from tension or trouble between man and wife. The quote from Erra suggests that sex can sometimes have negative results, as was the case with Anu having spawned the feared Sibitti demons.

Matters dealing with the toilet were also of interest to Anu-ikṣur as a possible cause of disease. He wrote a commentary on a therapeutic text and commented on the fact that a patient's tongue was swollen (Hunger 1976: No. 47, commenting on ibid. 46). Anu-ikṣur explained being swollen as being enlarged, associated with the "lurker-demon (*rābiṣu*) of the toilet." Anu-ikṣur then cited a proverbial hemerology (often quoted in antiquity), a text giving information about lucky and unlucky days of the month, which says that "if (the patient) enters the toilet (on that day), Šulak (the toilet-demon) will strike him" (*CAD* M/2 234; see Hunger 1976: No. 47, 15). Anu-ikṣur explained why: since he can etymologize Šulak's name as "(one having) unclean hands,"[201] therefore Šulak will strike one who enters a toilet with his unclean hands (Hunger 1976: No. 47, 4–5). Anu-ikṣur returned to this subject again, referring to dirt from a hole being from a refuse heap (possibly latrine), citing a proverbial phrase, "I poured dirt from a hole over my hand" (Hunger 1976: No. 50, 38–40). Without having the underlying text we cannot be sure of the context, but contact with dirt from the toilet suggests some awareness of the effects of poor hygiene.

Psychic causes

The recognition of physical symptoms having psychological dimensions is occasionally expressed in commentaries in a simplistic way. Another of Anu-ikṣur's commentaries refers to a man's speech changing[202] as a symptom of disease. The source text (from the Diagnostic Handbook Tablet 6) reports that a patient's "speech keeps changing and he continually wanders about" (Labat 1951: 64, 60′; Hunger 1976: No. 32, 8f.). Anu-ikṣur's comment on the passage reads, "delirium is usual for him" (Hunger 1976: No. 32, 9), giving a more precise explanation for "wandering about" in this context. Babylonian medicine was well aware of psychosomatic disease or disease resulting from mental illness (Stol 1999).

In this same commentary Anu-ikṣur explains what it means to find a man's voice sounding like the cry of an animal (probably a bird), with the prognosis being that the patient would die within a day (Hunger 1976: No. 32, 11; based on Labat 1951: 68, 87′). The commentary refers epigrammatically to a proverb: "death is the face of the Anzû(-storm)-bird," i.e. the potentially terrifying emblem of the god Ninurta (Hunger 1976: No. 32, 12). This cryptic comment is immediately explained: *an-zu-ú* : *an-šu-ú* : *i-šip-*[*pu*]; *anzû* (the bird) recalls the word for "dream interpreter"[203] who is a type of priest (*išippu*). The patient's voice was therefore altered by hysteria, perhaps as a result of a frightening vision or dream, comparable to seeing the terrifying Anzû-bird. Such brief comments or notes are suggestive of much more detailed discussion within the scribal schools.

The effect of demons is not ignored by commentaries when referring to disease. One commentary passage mentions that the patient's "feet [turn] inward, his shins turn inward," and Anu-ikṣur succinctly comments: "binder-demon" (Hunger 1976: No. 31, 34f.). In other words, the deformity referred to might be caused by a demon who "binds" magically, or a disease named after him. Why is this important medically? Because Anu-ikṣur associates a specific symptom with a specific cause, even if the cause is a term for a demon. This has to be distinguished, however, from magic, since medical texts and commentaries focus on specific symptoms caused by demons without considering other kinds of associated distress, as expressed in incantations.

Medical Terminology in Commentaries

More needs to be said about terminology within commentaries. Sometimes the word-for-word equations are asymmetric, which justifies our search for another level of meaning. One such equation is the Sumerogram sa.gig, which can be equated with an Akkadian loanword *sakikkū*, a general term for "symptoms" occasionally employed by the Assyrian Chief Physician Urad-Nanaya in his correspondence with Esarhaddon (Parpola 1993: Nos. 315, 320). Anu-ikṣur, in one of his commentaries, is thinking along the same lines and defines sa.gig as "all diseases" (*naphar murṣi*), referring potentially to any disease. Another Uruk medical commentary from one Šamaš-aha-iddin (perhaps a disciple of Anu-ikṣur) also defines sa.gig as "all diseases," but adds a more literal definition: "sore tendon."[204] Other learned commentaries, however, define the important logogram sa.gig in different ways. One unsigned commentary to Tablets 13 and 14 of the Diagnostic Handbook narrowly explains sa.gig as *kissatu*, a type of skin ailment (Dougherty 1933: No. 406, 17). Another commentary defines it as a more commonly attested disease, *maškadu*, a type of ailment associated with paralysis (see CAD M/1 368). Instead of the very limited definition of "sore tendon/sinew," or a definition based upon a specific condition, Anu-ikṣur offers a much broader definition embodied in the ancient name of the Diagnostic Handbook itself, namely *sakikkū*-symptoms. The student is being told to consider symptoms from all diseases as part of analogous thinking, rather than simply drawing conclusions from a local presentation of individual symptoms.

It is important to note how commentaries attempt to clarify vague symptoms. The fifth tablet of the Diagnostic Handbook concerns diseases of the eyes, mainly dealing with symptoms of the eyes, eyelids, eyeball, and all anatomy related to the eye. One passage can now be restored to read, "if his eyes are flayed, his lungs spit out his saliva and it flows from his mouth."[205] Anu-ikṣur explains this to mean that "he coughs and [expectorates] his phlegm" (Hunger 1976: No. 31, 31–2; based on Labat 1951: 50, 12). The general medical observation here is that coughing and expectorating are both associated with the lungs, but expelled in a different way from saliva dribbling from the mouth. Akkadian terminology is vague since there is no clear differentiation between "spittle," "mucous," and "phlegm" in the Akkadian medical thesaurus, which explains the focus of this commentary.

Fevers

One of the most difficult phenomena to explain in ancient medicine was the appearance of fever, either as a symptom or a disease in its own right. Without instruments or blood tests, an ancient physician had difficulty in distinguishing different types of fevers, except by rudimentary observations or noting regular patterns of the occurrence of fevers, spiking high temperatures punctuated by periods of cooling or chills. One such type of fever was *li'bu* (Stol 2007: 11–15), which we already encountered in commentaries on the Diagnostic Handbook, but the subject is elaborated in other Uruk commentaries as well. One commentary, probably from Anu-ikṣur (Hunger 1968: No. 30, with a damaged colophon), is based upon Tablet 4 of the Diagnostic Handbook dealing with symptoms associated with the temples of the head. The source text reads:

> If his (the patient's) temples, his epigastrium, and neck vertebrae constantly trouble (lit. "seize") him, and he shows no (signs) of low-grade fever or perspiration, by midday his pubic hair falls out, it is the Hand of Maiden Lilith, he is infected with *li'bu*-fever. (Labat 1951: 34, 20–1)

The first issue that concerned Anu-ikṣur is the relationship between the disease name ("Hand of Maiden Lilith") and the statement that the patient is "infected with *li'bu*-disease." To Anu-ikṣur's students, this connection may have been far from obvious. We have already encountered the picturesque disease terminology used by Babylonian medicine, often conferring upon diseases rather colorful names (usually "hand of" a god or demon), and such terminology can also be found in the early Hippocratic corpus (Geller 2004a: 20–1). Even if such disease nicknames were technical, they never completely lost the magical or religious connotations from the sphere from which they were derived.

The Hand of Maiden Lilith is a case in point, since there is a rich magical literature associated with this ghostly figure. She is the classic succubus who comes at night to seduce human males (or cause nocturnal emissions), because she died before puberty and the chance to have a lover or children. She was widely feared, although diseases labeled with her Hand were not necessarily transmitted sexually. Anu-ikṣur takes this matter up in his note explaining the verb *la'ābu*: "to be infected by *li'bu*-disease (means) the Lilû-demon spurned (or divorced) her" (Hunger

1976: No. 30, 7). This puzzling comment turns out to be an allusion to another text from Uruk archives, an incantation which refers in its opening to this Maiden Lilith escaping into the desert from the Lilû-demon who had chosen her (von Weiher 1983: No. 6, 1–3; Farber 1989a; Geller 2007: 213f. [= Ut. Lem. 5 183f.]). Anu-ikṣur gives a simpler version of this tale: the Lilû-demon spurned her. Being spurned and loveless is what made this demon so dangerous, although there is no explicit reason given by Anu-ikṣur to explain any connection with *li'bu*-disease; the relationship between a demon and disease often appears to us to be arbitrary.[206]

Once Anu-ikṣur's commentary has established that Maiden Lilith's personal predicament leads to infection, the next step is to define the disease itself more precisely. Anu-ikṣur tells us that "to be infected (*la'ābu*)" refers specifically to the disease *li'bu*, and the disease *li'bu* is synonymous with *ze'pu*, a word for a "mold" for casting metal objects, or later, a coin. Anu-ikṣur then elaborates on this equation in another of his commentaries, in which he associates the *ze'pu*-mold and *li'bu*-fever with *di-hu (di'u)*, "headache-fever" (Hunger 1976: No. 38, 10; see Stol 2007: 15–18, translating *di'u* as "malaria"). The question is how to distinguish *li'bu* from other kinds of fevers, such as ordinary "heat" (*ummu*) or "sun-fever" (*himiṭ ṣēti*). Anu-ikṣur's explanation employs the analogy of a *ze'pu*-casting mold or coin, which is hard on the surface but is associated with high levels of heat. The exact analogy between *li'bu*-fever and a casting mold are not clear, since this could refer to a description of the pathology of the fever or to an associated symptom, such as an abscess. Nevertheless, what is important is the logic of the commentary in which a fever is defined by processes outside the sphere of medicine.

Sometimes we find a commentary within a commentary. Tablet 13 of the Diagnostic Handbook contains a rather rare word, *hūṣu*, a type of stomach cramp: "if a patient cries, 'my stomach, my stomach!' he has stomach cramp (aṇd) internal distress – it is the Hand of Ištar" (Labat 1951: 126, 43). One commentary on this passages cites the word for stomach cramp (written *hu-uṣ-ṣa*), neatly defining it as "to roast, which is (also) to burn" (Dougherty 1933: No. 406, 10), and then adds another explanation: "Commentary and oral tradition on (the text) of 'if a patient's [right] hand [hurts him]' "; this latter phrase is the incipit of Tablet 11 of the Diagnostic Handbook (Labat 1951: 88, 1). The connection between these two different parts of the Diagnostic Handbook (Tablet 11 and 13) is far from obvious to us. However, what is more clear is that there is an attempt to define stomach cramps through an analogy of "roasting" or "burning" (*šamû, kabābu*), although neither of these terms appear elsewhere in medical literature. These are rather rare words drawn from cooking, which may not be coincidental. As Jacques Joanna points out:

> The fields from which Greek physicians drew visible evidence in order to deduce by analogy the internal functioning of the human body were quite varied, among them plants, animals, and arts; but cooking in the broad sense of the term remained the preferred field of reference. (Joanna 1999: 319)

The fact that a similar medical analogy was used by both Babylonian and Greek scholars is certainly worthy of note.

This same commentary also explains two words, *pāšittu* and *imtu*, although we cannot identify the exact passage in the Diagnostic Handbook from which they are taken. The first word, *pāšittu*, is a name of a female demon as well as a type of disease, characterized by symptoms of stomach pain and fever. The commentary adds: "*pāšittu* is that which contains bile" (Dougherty 1933: 406, 4). Although bile was a primary component of the Greek theory of humors, its role within Babylonian medicine is far from clear. Nevertheless, the commentary relates *pāšittu* to descriptions of disease in medical texts which refer to the patient vomiting bile. The second term, *imtu*, "poison" or even "spittle," adds another clue, since ancient scholarly glossaries also equate *imtu* "poison" with *martu*, "bile."[207] We may be dealing with a poison here, which is an aspect of Babylonian medicine hardly noted, although antidotes featured prominently in Greco-Roman medicine (Watson 1966). One reason for the lack of antidote recipes may have been that poisons were considered to belong to magic, like eating bewitched food, and therefore not the proper focus of medicine.

Physiognomy as diagnosis

Anu-ikṣur also took an interest in physiognomic omens, a branch of "medicine" (in a wider sense) in the ancient world, similar to diagnostic omens. Anu-ikṣur copied tablets of physiognomic omens, but he also wrote learned commentaries on such texts as well, much as he had done for diagnostic omens (Böck 2000: 99). In one case, Anu-ikṣur draws a medically relevant interpretation from a physiognomic omen predicting wealth and poverty:

> If a man has the head of a chameleon, and it is determined that he will be raised up (to wealth) but not collect (*šulû u la kaṣāru*), he will be impoverished and his inheritance [.....] (Böck 2000: 246)

Anu-ikṣur then comments:

> His wife will bend over for him,
> she will shrivel it up: as for his wife, he has not belittled her.
> (Sum.) "bir" = (Akk.) "shrivel" (*kalāṣu*).
> Alternative explanation: as for his wife, he can submit to her. (Böck 2000: 254)

We would interpret Anu-ikṣur's comments in the following way. The statement that "his wife will bend over for him" is intended for her to show him respect or offer him sex.[208] The next statement is surprising: "she will shrivel it up" probably refers to his penis.[209] Why is he impotent? The next phrase explains, "as for his wife, he has not belittled her."[210] Finally, Anu-ikṣur offers an alternative explanation: "as for his wife, he will submit to her."[211] The future of a man with a chameleon forehead is not rosy, since the predictions are that his family will abandon him and he will end up in poverty. The first explanation in the commentary is that his wife will be submissive to him, which may seem positive, but Anu-ikṣur then qualifies this meaning. He argues that actually the man will be submissive to her, resulting in his losing his sense of masculinity, unless he learns to put his wife in her place and take the upper hand. If not, he is doomed to suffer the fate predicted in the omen. In other words, Anu-ikṣur has altered the prediction, interpreting the man being "raised up" (*šulû*) to refer to his sexual potency, while the expression *lā kaṣāru* is interpreted as "not to bind" or restrict his wife, the combination of which will have bad results.

Iqīšâ

Anu-ikṣur was not the only Uruk scribe to write commentaries. A full and colourful Uruk medical commentary was probably composed by the prolific Uruk scholar, Iqīšâ, who lived some 75 years after Anu-ikṣur (see Robson 2008: 238; Hunger 1976: No. 13); the text is edited in full in the Appendix in this volume (Clay 1923: No. 32, cited hereafter as "Appendix"). Although the colophon of this tablet is damaged, one reason for ascribing it to Iqīšâ is because the commentary's source is a medical text from an Uruk tablet that belonged to this same Iqīšâ, according to its colophon (Thureau-Dangin 1922: No. 34; see Hunger 1968: No. 100).

We will limit our comments to various interpretations of medical texts. Iqīšâ's source text reads:

> If a man has stroke, epilepsy, Hand of the God-disease, (or) Hand of Ištar-disease,
> in order to get rid of it, its ritual is: take a male kid,
> recite into its right and left ears (the incantation) "An evil god, ditto"; you slaughter it. You take tears from the pupil of the eyes,[212] you take the *cover* of the cavities of head and neck (and) the fluid of its irises … (Thureau-Dangin 1922: No. 34: 1–5)

Early on in his commentary Iqīšâ explains the disease names, the first of which, "stroke,"[213] he reinterprets as follows: "the patient chokes and keeps spitting up phlegm" (see below, Appendix: 1). This is not a philological explanation but a medical one, since the general description of stroke in the Diagnostic Handbook mentions saliva (*ru'tu*) running from the patient's mouth (Labat 1951: 80, 2), but Akkadian *ru'tu* can refer to both "saliva" and "phlegm" (see Stol 1993: 8f.); Iqīšâ comments that a choking patient is likely to produce phlegm (or mucous) rather than saliva.[214]

Iqīšâ proceeds to explain the second disease name, often mentioned together with stroke, which is a type of "epilepsy" known by the rather poetic title of "Lord of the Roof."[215] Once again, our learned scholar defines this disease medically (avoiding any play on words): "'epilepsy' is (when) the right or left eye squints (lit. turns away)" (Appendix: 2; Stol 1993: 16). The phrase is actually a citation from physiognomic omens rather than medical literature, but in this case applied by Iqīšâ to describe a disease symptom.

We cannot identify the third-mentioned disease, the "Hand of the God"-disease, in modern terms, and this time Iqīšâ explains the nature of the disease ontologically by providing some background to the patient's medical history: "'Hand of the God'(-disease) (occurs when) the (patient) curses the gods, speaks blasphemy, (and) smashes whatever he finds" (Appendix: 2). In this case, the patient's disease is thought of as well-deserved divine retribution, and the expression "Hand of the God" is interpreted literally rather than metaphorically as a technical disease-name. The next disease on Iqīšâ's list is similar, known rather widely as the "Hand of Ištar"-disease, but in this instance the commentary gives a psychosomatic description of the patient's condition: "(the patient) keeps having stomach cramps (*huṣṣi*) and internal distress and he keeps forgetting his own words" (Appendix: 3).[216] None of these descriptions appears in the source text (Thureau-Dangin 1922: No. 34).

Iqīšâ also expounds the meaning of the "Hand of the Ghost," a common disease designation in Babylonian medical and magical literature. The commentary remarks that this condition occurs "(when) both (the patient's) ears ring, (a poultice) is *excessively applied*, (and) he cannot introduce his teeth to food" (Appendix: 3). The image of the ghost roaring into the patient's ears occurs frequently in therapeutic texts as a description of how the ghost can alter the patient's health, but this commentary is more specific. The patient loses all appetite and even lacks the strength to eat, which is a physical manifestation of what is essentially a psychic trauma caused by the attack of a ghost. In fact, Anu-ikṣur also comments on a similar passage in one of his commentaries based on a therapeutic text incipit: "if a man's ears roar through the attack of the Hand of a Ghost(-disease)," to which Anu-ikṣur comments: "his (ears) keep ringing ... the ghost has opened his ears."[217] Anu-ikṣur then puns on the word for ghost (*eṭemmu*) by etymologizing the word as the "one who gives an order" (*ṭēmu*), meaning that it is the ghost who is actually responsible for the patient's condition, rather than an abstract disease ascribed to a ghost on some remote grounds. A wandering unspecified ghost (*murtappidu, segû*) is actually responsible for causing the commotion, rather than the patient's being able to identify the ghost of a relative or ancestor who may be causing the difficulties (Stol 1993: 26).

Materia medica in commentaries

In this same commentary (see Appendix), Iqīšâ often embarks on explanations of *materia medica*, many of which are standard recipe ingredients. We find several drugs which can be classified as *Dreckapotheke*, which are usually disgusting or distasteful ingredients, but these turn out to be secret names of quite ordinary drugs, and the exotic names of these drugs were probably meant to discourage laymen from practicing medicine. In this way, "human semen" turns out to be a secret name for the very ordinary plant *maštakal* (see Appendix: 5), which occurs frequently in medical and magical contexts. A reference to "human skull" (presumably to be ground up) as *materia medica* turns out to be powder, while "human flesh" is a secret code for tamarisk, another common plant used in medicine (Appendix: 20). Other plants are not given secret names as such but employ colorful language to reflect interests in hygiene. One common resin, for instance, known as *abbukatu* is described as resembling "dust of a toilet" (Appendix: 14), which also appears as a medical substance in Talmudic medicine.

The common medicinal plant *kurkanû* is often described as "from the mountain" (hence imported), but in Iqīšâ's commentary *kurkanû* is also described as "being shaved like a crotch" (Appendix: 17); this may refer to the ritual shaving of a priest's entire body for purification purposes.

Many of the other references to *materia medica* in Iqīšâ's commentary are similar to those in many lists of medicinal plants and drugs, as well as in learned commentaries on them. Usually we find descriptions of the drugs rather than any real clues as to how they work, or what effects and side-effects these drugs were thought to have had upon the patient. In fact, we find a parallel literature, also known from late Uruk archives, in which the properties of plants and minerals are described in some detail (see von Weiher 1988: No. 106).

One drug in this particular commentary is described as a "panacea," for "any disease" (Appendix: 18), and the plant, *ašqulālu*, is described in rather cosmic terms as being "like an apple on the edge (or entrance) of the sea where there are neither plants nor reeds, growing on the surface of the waters" (Appendix: 18). Another plant, *azallû*, is described as a drug for "forgetting depression" (Appendix: 19), which suggests that it might have been popular in treating psychic distress or trauma, but in fact the drug appears commonly in potions and in salves for quite standard medical conditions, with little evidence that it was used to treat mental problems.

One drug is described in the commentary as "blood (kept) outside" (Akk. *kamû*), explained by Iqīšâ as "leper's blood," based on the idea that "outside" refers to a "leper" (Appendix: 7f.); a variant interpretation is "owl's blood."[218] The word for "blood" here (*dāmu*) often refers to the sap or juice of a plant, and in this case the juice (perhaps because of being toxic) is kept "outside" in a way analogous to a leper being kept outside the city, or like an owl (Appendix: 7–8).

In his commentary on the same base text, Iqīšâ explains the meaning of the rather cryptic *materia medica*, "canopy-hide" and "canopy-tendril":

> Hide of a canopy : black ox-hide which is from the western gate was worked into the top of the tamarisk (straps) of the canopy : tendrils : of the canopy : tendrils of tamarisk on top of which the black ox-hide was placed into the canopy. (Appendix 8–9)

Various parts of a canopy could be used with recipes, similar to a remark in the Babylonian Talmud that mattress ropes from a bed could also be used as *materia medica*.

Both Anu-ikṣur and Iqīšâ in their respective *oeuvres* comment on a physical feature of the medicinal plant *kukru*, describing a depression in the middle of the plant, while other aromatics were used as "cuttings" (Appendix: 14; Hunger 1976: No. 49, 31). It is not beyond the realm of possibility that Anu-ikṣur's teachings were still being taught in Uruk two centuries later.

Finally, Iqīšâ comments on a drug (*baluhhu*-resin) which is to be used by "one practicing medicine" (lit. "man of *asûtu*") (Appendix: 13). One might well presume that *all* drugs mentioned in medical texts could be used for medicinal purposes; so what is the point of this statement? However, Iqīšâ does not refer to the plant being used by an [lú]*asû*, but by a "man of healing" (lú *a-su-tu*$_4$), and this remark may point to the fact that *asûtu* was still recognized as a discipline, although the practicing *asû*-physician had virtually disappeared from view by Iqīšâ's day. In fact, Iqīšâ's commentary is about the latest reference to *asûtu* that we have, and the traditional distinction between *āšipu* and *asû* by this time had become virtually obsolete.

More Dreckapotheke

As mentioned above, commentaries and various lexical lists often include scholarly notes on *materia medica*. The plant lists, for instance, instead of describing a plant's or drug's properties, simply designate the disease for which it is most useful. Juniper (Akk. *burāšu*), for instance, is considered to be efficacious against jaundice (lit. "taboo"-disease, *ahhāzu*), as well as hepatitis, "gall"-related illnesses (perhaps referring to the gall bladder itself), and the disease *ašû*, as yet unidentified.

One plant, *nikiptu*, is glossed as "dog shit, dog's tongue, or dog's bone," all of which are varieties of *Dreckapotheke*.[219] What does this tell us about the plant's properties? The *Dreckapotheke* descriptions suggest something strong (feces) and moist (tongue), but also hard (bone), which by analogy summarizes the properties of this (as yet unidentified) plant or drug.[220] Iqīšâ's own commentary points out that the "male" variety of this plant is like tamarisk bark, compact and red, while the "female" variety is also like tamarisk bark, but thin and yellow-green (Appendix: 11–12). This plant is used regularly in prescriptions for salves and fumigation.

Another plant frequently commented upon is tamarisk, *bīnu*. Remarks appear in commentaries, e.g. "lion's blood" (*Dreckapotheke*) actually refers to juice from the middle of the tamarisk (CAD B 239). The description "lion's blood" may point to some characteristic of the drug itself, such as being "strong" or "potent." Another commentary gives a different view of tamarisk, describing it as having a wasteland habitat (*balītu*), although it is not the only plant to be described in this way (CAD B 63). This type of description may suggest a drying nature to the plant, since its habitat is associated with the steppe or wasteground.[221] The shoots of tamarisk are also listed in a vademecum as being effective against "Hand of the Oath"-disease (*BAM* 1 1 17).

Astrological medicine

One of the prominent principles of Greek astrological medicine was the theory of melothesia, which elaborated the influences of zodiac signs and individual planets over specified parts of the human anatomy and diseases. Although no Babylonian tablet deals with this kind of astral influence thematically, Reiner has discovered melothesia in a Late Babylonian medical commentary from Nippur, which resembles Uruk commentaries in being dictated by the *ummânu* as "questions and answers" (*maš'altu*) (Civil 1974: 336f.; Reiner 1993: 21f., 59f., 995). The entry which caught Reiner's attention is a learned comment on the typical medical phrases, "If a man's spleen hurts him" and "if a man's kidney hurts him." The commentary explains that the spleen is equated with Jupiter, and the "the Kidney-star is Mars" (Civil 1974: 336f.). Reiner correctly concludes that the intention of the commentary is to show that Jupiter governs the spleen and Mars governs the kidneys, which are clear examples of melothesia, as we know it from Greek sources. The late Nippur commentary serves as another example of how late commentary tablets provide fleeting glimpses into Babylonian medical theory, which often fails to appear elsewhere in the written record.

Writing Down of Medical Knowledge

By the time we get to late Uruk, the distinction between magic and medicine, and to a certain extent divination, is no longer valid. All of these scientific subjects have become integrated into a single scholarly curriculum, similar to the broadranging curriculum being developed in the Greco-Roman world (e.g. in Alexandria). The same scholars study the various genres, and the professional designations have virtually disappeared, except for that of the exorcist, who has become something of a philosopher (in the non-Greek sense).

We see evidence of late Uruk scribes classifying diseases, previously labeled as "Hand of a God," under generic disease-names without reference to divine causes. Second, a great interest emerged in late periods on writing commentaries, which reflected the discussions and lectures of the scribal schools, somewhat akin to what was happening in Aristotle's Lyceum. Although previously scribal curriculum concentrated on copying "set texts" – either the literary canon or received texts – there had been little interest in recording the wisdom of the *ummânu* or professor, whose insights and hermeneutics were intended to be learned orally and transmitted to the next generation of scholars. Although Babylonian scholars never adopted the habit, unfortunately, of actually writing down treatises and opinions on scientific matters (i.e. philosophy), nevertheless they began writing down notes or *Stichwörter* reflecting scholarly explanations of texts, including many medical texts. These commentaries can provide valuable insights into how received texts and ideas were being reinterpreted and adapted to changing conditions in Hellenistic Babylonia, and maybe to changing influences as well.[222]

To understand what was happening within Babylonian scholarship, it is helpful to look outside of Babylonia itself, to see what Plato had to say on the subject (Barton 1994: 134ff.). Plato makes an astute observation about the process of scientific learning:

> You might think that they [words] are speaking as if they were intelligent, but if you ask them something about what they have said, in the hope of learning, they just communicate the same thing for ever. (Barton 1994: 135)

In essence, Plato argues that there is a limit to what one can learn from a written text rather than through dialogue; one cannot question it, the text requires explaining, and one cannot become an autodidact based on a written text alone. The only legitimate learning comes from personal instruction, as Galen also insisted with his own students. As Barton says, "all the didactic texts of antiquity share the problem of communicating through the rigidity of the written form" (Barton 1994: 135). The same can be said for Babylonian scholarship, which was largely communicated through oral explanations of the *ummânu*, a small fraction of which were recorded in the form of commentary tablets.

One other aspect of Greek learning has Babylonian antecedents. As Plato again observes:

> Once it is written down, all speech circulates everywhere with no discrimination as to audience, equally among the wrong people, and it does not understand to whom it should speak, and to whom it shouldn't. (Barton 1994: 135)

A written document can fall into the hands of the initiated or ignorant, who misunderstand or misuse its contents, which is beyond the strict control of the master–student relationship. For this reason, scholarship was often treated as esoteric and not to be widely shared outside the small circle of adherents, as the astrologer Vettius Valens warned:

> I adjure you, most honoured brother, and all those being initiated into this systematic art ... to keep all these things hidden, and not to share them

> with the uninitiated, except those who are worthy to keep and receive them rightly. (Barton 1994: 136)

Barton explains such advice as originating in mystery cults, in which esoteric subjects such as astrology proliferated but were only intended to be taught to those initiated into the cult, who had taken an oath of allegiance. Such advice, however, is familiar from Babylonian colophons of scholarly tablets, which often declare that the tablet is to be shown only to those who are knowledgeable of the subject, rather than to those ignorant of it (Livingstone 1986: 260f.), and in fact we find an oath of allegiance being associated with those studying scholarly texts (such as divination) in Babylonia as well (Lambert 1998: 143).

These similarities in attitude to scholarship between the Babylonian and Greek worlds lend further support to the approach taken here, that "scribes" like Anu-ikṣur and Iqīšâ were in fact scholars in their own right, who were the authors of the commentaries which mention them by name. The likelihood of actual authorship is also supported by the number of commentary tablets ascribed to these scholars, since the very fact that we have so many commentary tablets mentioning Anu-ikṣur and Iqīšâ by name in colophons supports the argument in favor of the importance of these scholars as masters within the academy. Finally, the possibility that some of Anu-ikṣur's own hermeneutical comments may have been cited again two centuries later by Iqīšâ leaves open the prospect of scholarship being passed on through several generations of teachers, as certainly happened within Greek academies and schools.[223]

8

Medicine and Magic as Independent Approaches to Healing

Practice

The study of ancient Babylonian medical concepts and the persons who put them into practice gives us some useful insights into the art of healing. Medicine in the ancient world was a dynamic process, the result of an interaction between patient and therapist. It was understood that effective treatment of disease was not simply a matter of medical technology finding the right cure for the right illness. In a significant number of cases, the patient's own reaction to his being ill and to the treatment itself could affect the nature of the treatment and even help determine its success or failure. Of course we are only dealing with non-terminal disease in these instances, since many diseases were not necessarily fatal and could be improved by proper treatment. In any case, many non-fatal conditions are self-healing without or despite treatment.

One way of including the patient within the healing process was to use certain means which we would consider to be "magic." Since the normal reaction to the onset of disease is fear of death and anxiety about loss of health, magic harnessed various strategies to counteract these fears. These might include the therapist (in this case the exorcist) dressing up in a costume, as a fish-man or lion-man, and performing fumigations and rituals calculated to influence the patient's psychological state. If the patient's fears of the unknown could be focused on a specific object – such as a demon – magic could then be used to try to neutralize the patient's fear by offering effective anti-demonic rituals and incantations. On other occasions, if the patient felt a sense of guilt, which led him to believe that his illness was divine punishment for committing some transgression or violating some taboo, magic offered ritual penance through confession and appeals to divine mercy. If a patient was convinced that he was innocent but was being bewitched by an unknown rival or adversary, such psychosomatic illnesses could also be treated through appropriate recitation and ritual, in which icons of sorcery were burned or sent floating away in a boat. Such types of treatment (and many more) were recognized in Babylonia under a specific rubric, *āšipūtu*, "exorcism," but were incorporated into the healing processes.

At the same time, Babylonian science distinguished another form of therapy, *asûtu*, which we usually refer to as "medicine," although it was predominantly restricted to prescriptions of drugs. The boundaries between *āšipūtu* "exorcism" and *asûtu* "medicine" were permeable and not fixed, since medicinal remedies often included incantations and even rituals, borrowed from the sphere of magic, particularly as time went on. The further back we go into the history of Babylonian medicine, the more distinctive these two types of therapies appear to be. Early medicine contains no magic, and early magic contains no medicine, as far as the limited evidence available allows us judge. Throughout the second millennium BC, the exorcist and physician maintained separate realms of activity, with relatively little overlap. By the advent of the first millennium BC, incantations increasingly embodied short rituals which resembled medicinal remedies, while at the same time medical prescriptions included more and more magic. However, just as magic rituals and medical recipes were still distinctive, magical and medical incantations also differed from each other. Magical rituals tended to use fumigation and external applications of magical concoctions, while medical prescriptions favored potions and ingesting of drugs, as well as pessaries and suppositories.[224] On the other hand, magical incantations tended to be elaborate formal recitations involving healing gods advising about effective remedies, while medical incantations look more like folk magic, usually simple doggerel poetry or even mumbo-jumbo spells which were no longer understood. The genres of magic and medicine, therefore, were relatively distinct and unmistakable.

The professions that practiced magic and medicine are equally distinguishable in our sources. Looking back at archives from the second millennium BC, we find abundant documentary evidence for the *asû*-physician dominating the field of medicine, with hardly a reference to the activities of exorcists. However, the disjuncture in our source material from this period is hard to explain, since at this very time we find a great many incantations but precious few medical prescriptions. By the first half of the first millennium BC, the respective roles of physician and exorcist are still recognizable, although it is becoming clear that exorcists are gaining ground within the sphere of medical expertise. Private libraries of exorcists reveal an interest in many kinds of medical treatments as well as traditional incantations, and at the Assyrian royal court both the Chief Physician and Chief Exorcist wielded considerable influence. Colophons of tablets in the seventh century BC still distinguish between *asûtu* and *āšipūtu*. Nevertheless, changes occurred after the Persian conquest of Babylonia by Cyrus which appear to have caused seismic changes in how health care was delivered from that time on. Probably modeled on the influence and interests of the magi, Babylonian exorcists gradually take over the practice and study of magic and medicine from this time on, and in many ways the exorcists appear to dominate the intellectual scene in Hellenistic Babylonia. They were expected to have knowledge of divination, astrology, lexicography, medicine, and magic, judging by colophons of late tablets and the professional interests of the scribes who copied them (Robson 2008: 258–60).

These changes in status of exorcist and physician did not cause major changes in how magic and medicine were practiced in late periods, as far as we are able to tell. Traditional bilingual incantations known from the second millennium BC were still being copied in the Hellenistic period by scholars from Babylon and Uruk, such as Tanittu-Bēl and Iqīšâ. Medical texts were recopied in their traditional form, with at least two important innovations. One, astral magic and astral medicine began to become popular, especially in Babylon, taking advantage of great advances in astronomical knowledge which emerged in the Persian period, after c. 500 BC. The ability of astronomers to predict celestial events made a deep impression on scholars in other disciplines, and attempts were made to adopt the same methodology in trying to predict the course of disease, by drawing analogies with celestial predictions. Hence, illnesses developing under a certain zodiacal sign might be influenced by the course of the constellation (Barton 1994: 189). This keen interest in astronomy and astrology altered some ancient views on medicine, since astronomers were able to comprehend the movements of stars without referring to any divine plan or agency, and this had a profound effect on ancient thinking, even in Babylonia.

Our attempt to follow the interests and careers of exorcists, doctors, and even patients within Babylonian medicine has not been straightforward, since the ancient evidence is multifaceted and unevenly distributed between various periods of Babylonian history. We have also encountered some problems which are difficult to unravel, mostly surrounding the complex relationships between medicine and magic in Babylonia, and we have seen how this relationship changed substantially over the course of time. We cannot expect either ideas or professions to remain static over a period of some two millennia, although changes themselves can be difficult to document. Nevertheless, the fortunes of healers and their patients within society and progress in medical thinking are fundamental aspects of ancient medicine, and it is crucial to document these developments in order for Babylonian medicine to take its rightful place within the history of the subject.

Theory

The distinction between "medicine" and "magic" can be detected in the physical layout and format of the cuneiform tablets themselves, which any trained Assyriologist can recognize at twenty paces. Magical texts usually contain long incantations and short rituals, while medical texts usually contain long or large numbers of recipes (corresponding to the magical rituals) and short incantations. As always there are exceptions, but in general other distinctive characteristics help us identify an incantation from a medical text. Incantations usually begin with the word *šiptu* "incantation" in the form of its Sumerogram én, and likewise an incantation often ends with a Sumerian rubric labeling it as an incantation (ka-inim-ma) or as a spell (tu_6.én), or both. Rituals appended to incantations tend to be brief, and rituals bear their own labels indicating a ritual belonging to an incantation. In most cases, the incantation itself is the primary text with an appended ritual belonging to the incantation.[225] Medical texts, on the other hand, have a different format, framed by a casuistic structure typical of legal texts and omens. Each individual section (sometimes only a single line, or several lines ruled off) usually begins with the phrase, "If a man (suffers from)" a certain ailment, followed by a listing of the *materia medica* of a recipe, then closing on an optimistic note that the patient will get better.[226] No ancient scribe would confuse the following medical text for an incantation:

> If a man suffers from dribbling urine,
> he should keep drinking one *sila*-measure of
> ash of the hoof of a spring lamb,
> one *sila* of ash of male mandrake
> on an empty stomach in water for five days;
> he should keep drinking throughout the day and he will get better. (*BAM* 7 1: 10′–13′)

In some cases, recipes are accompanied by brief incantations with typical incantation rubrics, although it is clear that recipes are primary while the incantations are secondary.

There are actually several different types of incantations found within the contexts of either "magic" or "medicine." First, there are Sumerian unilingual incantations, many of which go back ultimately to the third millennium or Old Babylonian period (Cunningham 1997: 80–6; Schramm 2008; van Dijk & Geller 2003). These are often *Kultmittelbeschwörungen*, incantations to purify various items used in the temple cult or for healing rituals. The next phase of incantation literature introduced Sumerian–Akkadian bilingual incantations, which was a tradition which endured well into the first millennium BC. These consisted of rather formal incantations which included the traditional dialogue between powerful deities taking an interest in the patient's plight (Falkenstein 1931: 53–8; Cunningham 1997: 79f., 120f.). A third category of incantations were Akkadian only. These often dealt with scorpion stings, snakebite and dog-bite (Finkel 1999), or incantations against rivals.[227] Other genres of "folk magic" exist in both Sumerian unilingual and Akkadian unilingual versions, but not bilingual texts, such as love incantations and so-called "evil eye" incantations (see Cunningham 1997: 105, 111; Geller 2004). These are not the types of incantations which appear within the medical corpus, as appended to therapeutic recipes. A clear distinction in both form and content can be made between incantations within the corpus of magic and those within a corpus we define as medicine.

Furthermore, there is the matter of terminology. On one hand, it is correct to say that neither Sumerian nor Akkadian has specific words for either "magic" or "medicine," but this does not tell the whole story, since other kinds of terminology are certainly relevant to the discussion. Aside from making a distinction between two types of healers, the "exorcist" (*mašmaššu* or *āšipu*)[228] and "physician" (*asû*), Akkadian texts distinguish between two types of associated professional literature, *mašmaššūtu/āšipūtu* and *asûtu*, indicating the studies of exorcism and medical therapy, as practiced by the two professions. At the same time, Akkadian recognizes a word for "black arts" or "witchcraft" (*kišpu*), which is a general term for the wrong kind of magic, for which the associated professionals, "(male) witch" (*kaššapu*) and especially the "(female) witch" (*kaššaptu*) are well known (see Schwemer 2007: 69–158). This is typical for Mesopotamia, whose languages usually express abstract ideas in a more concrete form than in corresponding European languages, such as Greek or Latin. In this guise, the term *mašmaššūtu/āšipūtu* and *asûtu* denote "magic arts" and "healing arts," referring to the actual crafts of writing and using texts devoted to exorcism and therapeutic recipes, or in more abstract terms, "magic" and "medicine."[229]

The point is that if one rejects the distinction between "magic" and "medicine" in Mesopotamia, it becomes difficult to explain the different roles adopted by these two professionals, as well as their respective orientations. It appears that private tablet archives or libraries belonging to exorcists contained medical texts as well (Jean 2006), which raises difficult questions regarding the difference between the exorcist's training and that of the *asû*-physician. Does this also mean that the physician would have studied the art of exorcism as well as drug therapy during the course of his training? Would he have been responsible for composing incantations found within medical texts, or would he have relied upon the exorcist to supply these for him? If either of these professionals could work on his own, without the other, why is the duplication of roles necessary, desirable, or even practical, persisting as it did over so many generations?[230]

If, on the other hand, we accept this basic distinction between magic and medicine, some things become clear. The first relevant point here is that the *mašmaššu* and *asû* would have had very different orientations in regard to disease. The exorcist, for one thing, would have been concerned with a much broader range of issues than ill-health, since his incantations had to deal with every aspect of a person's relationship to the gods. Angry gods, moreover, could potentially bring all kinds of misfortune, as well as ill-health. The exorcist also acted as religious consultant in his basic role as priest, and would have been expected to know much more about the cosmos than was required by healing or medicine. For instance, the *mašmaššu* would have been expected to know about witchcraft and how to counteract it, in all its many forms. He would have to know about the workings of all kinds of demons. He needed to know about omens and what spells were required to counteract bad portents, such as *namburbî*-omens (see Maul 1994). He would have to know about spells against impotence and other spells to attract a lover, or counter-charms against gossip and rivals. He would have to be familiar with rituals and incantations concerned with inaugurating a new cult idol (Shibata 2008: 193f.). All such matters were part of his large repertoire.

Nevertheless, the exorcist played a crucial role in medicine and healing because no other misfortune which can strike is quite the same as illness. Everyone is affected by illness at some time or another, or at least someone close is affected by it. Of all possible calamities, illness is certainly the most common, and for this reason most of the exorcist's arsenal of incantations were devoted to illnesses, either psychic or physical.

This is probably one reason why it is the exorcist who makes the medical prognosis or diagnosis, based upon his experience of dealing with illness as a dominant form of human suffering.

The *asû*, on the other hand, has no other role to play outside of medicine. From our very limited understanding of the full range of his tasks, we assume that his concern was primarily with drugs and drug-related therapies, and not much else. This already shows us an important difference in orientation between these two professionals. Whether the *asû* may also have treated wounds is impossible to say, although it is conceivable that some other semi-professional (Akk. *gallābu*, comparable to the medieval barber-surgeon) operated on patients, but left no written record of his activities or techniques.[231]

The more significant difference between *mašmaššu* and *asû* has to do with their respective intellectual approaches to illness and healing. The exorcist's working assumption was that gods determine man's destiny and illness is ultimately a manifestation of this fact. Therapy, according to the exorcist, must always take this into account, first and foremost. The practice of "medicine" (*asûtu)*, although subscribing to this same notion, was orientated towards the more immediate problem of treating symptoms, such as pain, fever, or vomiting, with palliative drugs or similar types of remedies. The role of the gods in these matters was largely secondary. The approach of the *asû* was not necessarily more "rational" than that of the exorcist, since much of the physician's healing repertoire no doubt consisted of placebo drugs or those that simply had no effect. Nevertheless, one way of understanding the difference between *mašmaššu* and *asû* can be described as "magic" versus "medicine," that is competing systems of healing in which the patient's relationship to the divine played a more prominent role in one system, but hardly any role in the other.

Appendix: An Edition of a Medical Commentary

The following text is an edition of a commentary as an example of the genre, since the text was last edited some 85 years ago (Campbell Thompson 1924), probably composed by the Uruk scholar Iqīšâ, who flourished in the latter part of the fourth century BC. Many items from it are discussed above. Several texts have thus far been identified as the source texts for this commentary, the main one being Thureau-Dangin 1922 (=TCL 6): No. 34, with duplicates. The source text is partly edited and translated below.

Clay 1923 (= BRM 4): No. 32 = MLC 1863

Top edge (not copied, read from photo): *ina a-mat* ^{d}*anu* ^{d}*an-ti* ^{d}*be-let-ni* ^{d}kù.sù *u* ^{d}nin-girimma *liš-lim*

1 si.dara$_{4}$.maš[232] : *qar-nu a-a-lu* : si : *qar-nu* : dàra.maš : *a-a-lu* : diš : *šum-mu* : an.ta.šub.ba[233] : *mar-ṣa ih-tan-naq ù* úh-*su* šub.šub-*a* : an.ta.šub.ba

2 ^{d}lugal.nir.ra : igi^{II} 15-*šú u* 150-*šú i-kap-pi-iṣ*[234] ^{d}lugal.nir.ra : šu.dingir.ra : dingir.meš *i-nam-zar šil-lat i-qab-bi šá im-mar i-mah-haṣ* šu.dingir.ra : šu. ^{d}innin.na :

3 *hu-uṣ-ṣi* gaz šà tuk.tuk-*ši ù* inim.meš-*šú im-ta-na-áš-ši* šu.^{d}innin.na : šu.gedim. ma geštug^{II}.meš-*šú* gù.dé.meš *ma-gal iṭ-ṭè-né-pi šin-na-šú ana ma-ka-le-e*

4 *la ú-qar-ra-ba-ma* šu.gedim.ma : dù.dù.bi : *e-pu-uš-ta-šú* : *nap-šar-šú ú-ru-di* su : *ta-a* : *a-pir* : *hu-up-pat*$^{!}$: *šup-lu-šú* : *šup-lu* : *a-pir šá* sag.du

5 *u* gú[235] : ì hul : *nap-ṭu u* ì ku$_{6}$[236] : *šam-ni nu-ú-nu* : a.ri.a nam.lú.lu$_{18}$.lu[237] : ^{ú}*maš-ta-kal* : *áš-šú* ^{ú}a.ri.a : ^{ú}*maš-ta-kal šá-niš* a.ri.a : *ri-hu-ut* :

6 túg.níg.dára : *ú-la-pi* : šu.lál : *lu-up-pu-ut-tu*$_{4}$: túg.níg.dára šu.lál : uzu ka$_{5}$.a : ^{ú}*tara-muš* : *ki-ma* suhuš ^{ú}*si-il-qa* : ú.igi-*lim ki-ma* gìr.pad.du nam.lú.u$_{18}$.lu

7 : ^{ú}igi-a ia ^{d}15 ani ^{ú}igi-a ia ú.^{d}utu numun- ia ii (sic) : múd aii : múd lú aaban a :

8 lú aaban ni múd[238] ad ^{mušen} : diš-ni : ia : in ii aa hi.hi : hi.hi : baa : ^{zì}še.muš$_5$: i pp : kuš and $_5$-i [239] :

9 kuš gu$_4$ .a ina abul uru im.mar.tu ina i giš.šinig and $_5$-i innpp : ia : and $_5$-i : ia giš.šinig kuš gu$_4$ .a ana and $_5$-i

10 ina i ana : máš.zu[240] : ii : máš : i .a : zu : d : aà hab : naaa : ia baa . .a : ú.tilla ia giš.šinig sa$_5$:

11 ú.lú-^{d}an : ia aa ibi : ú.aš : ia aa tu.mušen : šim.an.bar nita ia ip giš.šinig a .a sa$_5$ niip mí ia ip giš. šinig

12 aa a : peš$_{10}$.^{d}íd : úh.^{d}íd[241] : peš$_{10}$.^{d}íd : a $_4$: peš$_{10}$.^{d}íd : a.gar.gar.^{d}íd : peš$_{10}$.^{d}íd .aiind

13 peš$_{10}$.^{d}íd ba.ba.za.^{d}íd : peš$_{10}$.^{d}íd p . $_4$: mun eme.sal.lim : mun bbi íd : illu ^{šim}buluh ii ana lú a $_4$ innp : illu li.dur

14 : ia pi a : ^{šim}hab : .i : ina : ibii : ^{šim}gúr.gúr pp bb ú ^{šim}bulug šim.meš.la[242] ^{šim}gúg.gúg[243] : ^{šim}mug[244] šim.šal

15 ibii ina šú.^{d}utu e- [245] šim.hi.a : [246] : abana $_4$: ^{giš}eren sumun : pi : ^{giš}eren sumun ni ba .ii $_4$[247] šà ^{giš}eren : ^{mun}aan ù.mu.un : aan

16 [ù.m]u.un da mun aa kur adaaa : im.sa$_5$: : ^{ú}an ia a $_4$ b ^{ú}an dii

17 [^{ú}na] : ^{ú}an a aa ^{ú}apaina : ì.giš bur : ì.giš bara$_4$: biiii : bur : biiii ani ì.nun.na ai ì a .a ibii

18 [............] x x ma : napa . : ^{ú}lal[248] : ia ^{giš}hašhur ina ni a i aa a ^{giš}gi a ba ina igi a.meš è ina i

19 [................................] x x aa an i : ^{ú}a.zal.lá : ia ^{ú}ana sa$_5$: ú.a.zal.lá : ú niia a : ú.kur.kur :

20 [..] x zi ibi b : band [249] : nam.lú.u$_{18}$.lu : giš.šinig : uzu nam.lú.u$_{18}$.lu

21 [...] x x appai : ia : paa .a$^{!}$-n [250] lú.bappir ana idi še.bar gazi.sar diš-ni hi.hi-a

22 [...] ú$^{?}$ suhuš giš.šinig è- ni a n giš.šinig : $^{\text{na4}}$ab - : $^{\text{na4}}$ab

23 [..] x pa : pi appia ana igi- apaa : ap :

24 [.................................] ú$^{?}$ bai : ^{ú}har.lum.ba.šir a i . ni $_4$: ú.ia

25 [...] x : ^{ú}aaniia : ^{ú}a ni $_4$

26 [...] : ^{ú}ku$_6$: a n n aaaan

27 [...] x sar : ú ppa $_4$: ú ban

28 [.. bi] aa : aabi : a ![251] kur ba ki [...]

29 [...] ú x x nu x ia pi šah :

30 rest broken

1 [........................ n apa]- ib (e pi

2 [........................ lúumbisag-n a -da-n] -dn a m (numun)-iiii (hé.giš)[252]

3 [... pai a]n an - ! iabba (tùm)-

4 [253]x .meš- abi i im é.abzu : numun? úka.zal ip . .a-ni $_4$[254] : abba : inai ban[255] geštugII aabi

5 úpa - $_4$a . : úka.tar : dím.ma.an.ta : áš- $_4$[256] tuk-i : ú pa gi zú.lum.ma sumun : b .iin dii

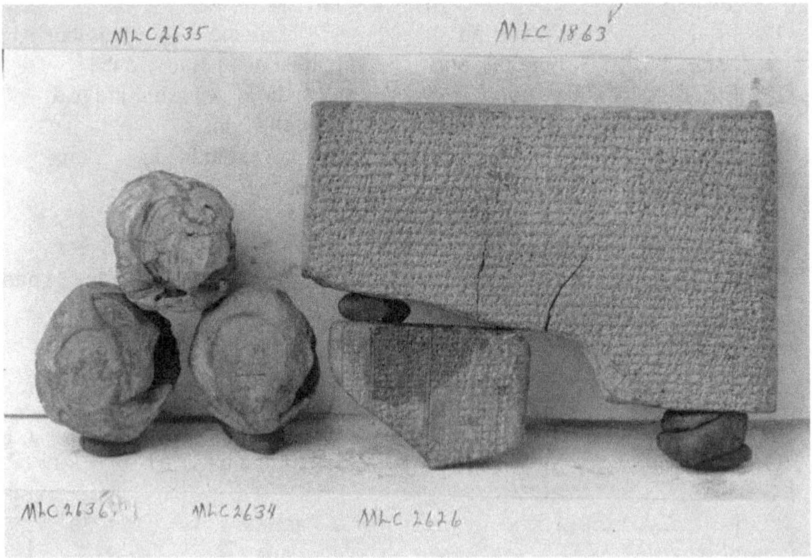

igureA.1 Photo of MLC 1863 taken by A.T. Clay (photo courtesy Ulla Kasten, Yale Babylonian Collection)

ranslation

1 (The term) "stag's horn" (Sum.) is translated by "stag's horn" (Akk.);[257] "horn" (Sum.) is translated by "horn" (Akk.); "stag" (Sum.) is translated by "stag" (Akk.). (The term) "if" (Sum.) is translated by "if" (Akk.). The term "stroke" (Sum.) indicates that the patient chokes and keeps spitting up phlegm; "stroke" (Sum.) (and)

2 "epilepsy" (Sum.) is (when) the right or left eye squints (lit. turns away). "Hand of the God(-disease)" (occurs when) the (patient) curses the gods, speaks blasphemy, (and) smashes whatever he finds; "Hand of the God" (also) refers to "Hand of the Goddess,"

3 and (occurs when the patient) constantly has stomach cramps and "heart-ache" and keeps forgetting his words. "Hand of the Goddess" (also) refers to "Hand of the Ghost(-disease)," (when) both (the patient's) ears ring, (a poultice) is i appid , (and) he cannot introduce his teeth to food.

4 Hand of the Ghost(-disease): "its ritual" (Sum.) is translated by "its ritual" (Akk.). His uvula is the body's windpipe. (The word) "cover" means "covered." The "cavity" refers to its "depression," the "depression" is (what is) "covered by the head

5 and neck." "Naptha" (Sum.)[258] is translated by "naptha" (Akk.), and "fish oil" (Sum.) is translated by "fish oil" (Akk.). Human sperm (Sum.) is the same as (the plant) aaa , which is derived from "steppe-plant."[259] A second explanation for aaa is "semen" (Sum.), which is the same as "semen" (Akk.).[260]

6 (The term) "towel" (Sum.) is translated by "towel" (Akk.); "soiled" (Sum.) is translated by "soiled" (Akk.).[261] "Soiled towel" (Sum.) is the same as "fox flesh." (The plant) aa is like the root of beetroot.[262] i -plant is like human bone.[263]

7 a -plant is like a lunar radiance;[264] another (meaning): a -plant is like a sunflower, its seed is like barley. Blood (kept) outside[265] means leper's blood; semantically "outside" (can refer to)

8 a leprous man; another meaning is blood of an owl. "Together" means "when" one is mixed with one another. "Mix" (Sum.) is "to mix" (Akk.). (Sum.) še.muš$_5$ is (Akk.) -barley, a late(-growing) cereal. "Hide of a canopy" refers to a

9 black ox-hide which is from the western gate, worked into the top of the tamarisk (straps) of the canopy. Tendrils (referring to) the canopy are tendrils of tamarisk on top of which the black ox-hide was

10 placed into the canopy.[266] (Male) goat (Sum.) is translated by (male) goat (Akk.); a goat (Sum.) is translated by goat (Akk.), and "zu" (Sum.) means "familiar."[267] "Smelly plant" means "you remove it," like sand. (The plant) . is like tamarisk and red.

11 (The plant) a a n is like the dung pellet of a raven. “Single”-plant is like the dung pellet of a dove. Male niip -plant is like tamarisk bark, firm and red, while female niip -plant is (also) like tamarisk bark,

12 but thin and yellow-green. -sulphur is green sulphur, aaa - sulphur is black sulphur,

13 pappa -sulphur is white sulphur. a -salt refers to salt from mid-river. a -resin is resin which is used by a “man of healing (a).” Aba -resin is

14 like the dust of the latrine.[268] (The plant) šim.hab (Sum.) is translated by . (Akk.). (The plant) ina is (used as) cuttings. -plant) (is characterized) by depressions in the middle of the plant, (while) ba (-plant), ia (-plant), (-plant), (also) equal na (-plant) and i a are (all)

15 cuttings which come out in the evening. Aromatic-plants ( ) are the same as aromatics (Sum.) are the same as frankincense. Eren.sumun (Sum.)[269] is the same as p .[270] Eren.sumun has a second explanation, a beetle which inhabits the cedar-tree.[271] Aa n -salt is

16 ù.mu.un (Sum.) and is the same as aa n ,[272] ù.mu.un (Sum.) is (also) blood because the salt of Media is red. “Red clay” (Sum.) is a “red clay” (Akk.). n (-plant) is like a shaved crotch, a n (-plant) of the mountain.

17 a (-plant) is the same as a n of the land (and) is the same as the apaina (-plant). Oil of a p (-vessel)[273] is the same as pressed oil (Sum.)[274] (since) a bii -(stone jar) is the same as a p (-vessel). (Oil of) a bii - (stone jar) has another explanation, (namely) “ghee,” a third explanation is “pressed oil,” and a fourth explanation is

18 [...........]... A panacea[275] is the aa -plant (Sum.), (which is) like an apple-tree, it grows in reclaimed (dirt) of the sea where there is neither plant nor reed, (and) on the surface of the water, and above which is

19 [................................] (is used for) a childbirth clyster.[276] The aa (-plant) is like the ana (-plant) and is red. The aa (-plant) is an anti-depressant drug.[277] (The plant) aai is

20 [.......................................].. a .[278] d is (given as) “human skull,” tamarisk is (given as) “human flesh.”[279]

21 [...]...of the marsh is ia ,[280] which are brewer’s grindings, (which) you mix together into a cereal of barley and a and

22 [..]The plant which grows from the tamarisk root has another explanation: tamarisk moss is (also) alum.[281] Alum is

23 [...] An ape is a monkey whose snout bends back towards his face: “turned back” is

24 [..................................] Subarean-plant is an (-plant), a drug (against) stricture. ia (-plant) is

25 [...]... Aania (-plant) is (the same as) a n (-plant).

26 [...] slag is also a n (-plant), literally “fish plant.”[282]
27 [...] a (type of) “thicket-plant” is papyrus.
28 [..] A “caterpillar” is (also) a “dormouse,” also to be explained as a “nobody from Subartu.”[283]
29 [...]........ like burning (is a) pig :
30 [................

(colophon)

1 [............................who is] wise and whose speech
2 [......., So-and-So son of So-and-so,] astrologer, descendant of Zer-kitti-lishir
3 [...................................One who fears] Anu and Antu will not carry it off.

ain in ab

4 Soft .... of the clay of the Eabzu-temple, seed of aa -plant), and in ip (-plant) : he “softens” means he “cuts.” The “bow” of the ears of a dormouse. A fast-working thicket-plant. Fungus is “fashioned from heaven”(-plant) means he has what he needs. Drug, frond, reed, old date: bid n is “lamp of the mountain”(-plant).

he Sourceext

The source text for the above commentary is contained in TCL 6 34, with the following duplicates: BAM 178; AMT 35,3, and BAM 388 i 9 (Babylonian script, provenance unknown); and BAM 179. Only TCL 6 34 is edited below with appropriate restorations from duplicate sources.

1 [diš an.t]a.šub.ba ^{d}lugal.ùr.ra šu.dingir.ra šu.^{d}innin.na
2 [ana] lú gál-i ana zi-i dù.dù.bi máš.zu ti-
3 [ina ge]štug^{II}- 15 150 én n min šid-n kud-i
4 [é]r lamma- igi-i[284] aa pa sag.du gú
5 a.meš gi$_6$ igi^{II}- ti- ì hul ì ku$_6$ múd giš.erin
6 ^{ú}ina.uš numun ^{ú}ina.uš múd ^{mušen}adii kuš and $_5$-i

7 ia and $_{5}$-i a (kù.gi dadag.meš ^{ú}aa ^{ú}igi-i ^{ú}igi-a
8 [súd hi.h]i gu$_{7}$- nag- šéš- ina dè sar-a tin- .
9 [14 ú.hi.a] a (gur) máš.zu

---

10 [.................] x x ^{ú}tilla ^{ú} lú -an
11 (trace)

. ii

1 $^{\text{na4}}$ab gìr.pad.du n[am.lú.u$_{18}$.lu
2 si dara$_{4}$.maš KA.a.ab.ba gìr.p[ad.du ....
3 14 ú.hi.a a (gur) x [....

---

4 $^{\text{na4}}$ab gìr.pad.du nam.lú.u$_{18}$.lu [...
5 ^{ú}aa gìr.pad.da pi (ugu.dul.bi) x [...

---

6 ^{giš}alan$^{?}$.a ú x x x [...........

. iii

1 x x x [...
2 ^{ú}.a .n ú si sik šá x[.....

---

3 muš.dím.gurun.na u$_{5}$.meš edin[285] li šini[g]
4 ^{ú}ana ^{ú}kur.kur peš$_{10}$.^{d}íd ^{zì}buru$_{5}$.habrud.d[a]
5 hénbur ^{giš}má an šinig 10 ú.hi.a a (kù.gi) gaz bbi
6 ^{ú}ana ^{ú}kur.kur naga.si ina dè sar- a kù.gi) gaz bbi
7 múd buru$_{4}$.ge$_{6}$ ^{mušen} $^{\text{na4}}$zálag ^{ú}in$_{6}$-b $_{17}$-ai ^{ú}n .ab
8 ^{giš}šur.mìn ^{ú}pa ^{nim}ur.gi$_{7}$ ppa ib a.šà
9 sahar dal.ha.mun sahar sila.lím.ma ^{ú}lú.u$_{18}$.lu šinig
10 15.ú.meš napa gaz bbi

---

11 1 gín ^{ú}aa gín ^{ú}igi-i 4- ^{ú}igi-a 1 g[ín šinig[286]]
12 1 gín ^{ú}ina.uš gín ^{ú}úkuš 1 gín ^{ú}a
13 gín KA.a.ab.ba 1 gín apa ann 1 gín numun ^{giš}ha.lu.úb
14 1 gín ^{ú}n 2 gín ^{ú}har.har 1 gín [^{ú}l]uh.mar.tu
15 1 gín nu.luh.ha gín ^{ú}kur.kur 1 gín šim.[......................]
16 gín ^{giš}šul.hi 1 gín numun šinig pap [............................]

. i [287]

1 (traces)
2 [.................................]ur.gi$_{7}$

3 [.................................] x du
4 [...........................] x p -p
5 [.........................] ^{ú}ku$_6$ šinig
6 [.............................] x úkuš.hab
7 [........................] ^{ú}gír ^{giš}
8 [..................] ^{ú}aana $_4$ ^{na4} .a
9 [^{na4} peš$_{10}$].^{d}íd úh.^{d}íd a.gar.gar.^{d}íd
10 [ba.ba.za ^{d}íd ^{giš}]a -a ^{giš}eren.sumun ^{giš}šur.mìn
11 [^{giš}gír ^{šim}]man.du ^{šim}li ^{šim}gúr.gúr ^{šim}gig ^{šim}šeš
12 [niip] nita mí ^{giš}še.ná.a a.ri.a nam.lú.u$_{18}$.lu
13 [app šah .]p gu$_4$ baia na -
14 [pap] 19 ú.hi.a napa kúm

---

15 [...] x ^{ú}kur.kur ^{ú}igi-i ^{ú}igi-a li šinig ^{ú}hur.sag
im.1.kam a (kù.gi) igi.tab
16–18 Colophon, cf. Hunger 1968: No. 100

Translation of ll. 1–9

1 [If] stroke, epilepsy, Hand of the God-disease or Hand of the Goddess-disease
2 befall a man, in order to remove it, its ritual (is): you take a male kid,
3 you recite [in] its right and left ear the incantation, "Evil ditto"; you slaughter (it).
4 You take tears from the pupil of the eyes and the of the depressions of the head and neck,
5 (and) fluids of its irises, naphtha, fish oil, cedar-"blood,"
6 aaa , aaa -seed, owl blood, hide of a canopy,
7 tendril of a canopy – (all) pure fumigants; you crush and mix aa ii and ia -plants,
8 you have him drink and eat (them), you anoint him and fumigate him over ashes and he will recover.
9 [14 drugs for the] fumigation of a male kid.
10 [.......] . -plant, "man-like"-plant.

. ii

1 Alum, human bone [....
2 stag's horn, coral, bone [.....
3 14 drugs for fumigation of ..[..................

---

4 Alum, human bone [...
5 aa , monkey-bone, ..[........

. iii

3 Copulating geckos of the steppe, juniper, tamarisk,
4 an , aai , sulphur, partridge,
5 sprout of a boat, cumin, tamarisk, 10 drugs for fumigation for "heartache."
6 You fumigate him with an , aai , and alkali in cinders; fumigation for a "heartache."
7 Blood of a black raven, shiny stone, coral, n .ab ,
8 cypress, pa -juniper, "dog"-fly, mole-cricket of the field,
9 dust of the storm, dust of crossroads, a a n -plant, tamarisk,
10 15 drugs as a salve for "heartache."

---

11 aa , half shekel ii , a quarter (shekel) of ia 1 shekel [tamarisk]
12 1 shekel aaa half shekel cucumber, 1 shekel a ,
13 half shekel coral, 1 shekel aann -turnip, 1 shekel seed of .-tree,
14 1 shekel mint, 2 shekels a , 1 shekel ^ú ibba ,
15 1 shekel n , half shekel aai , 1 shekel ..[.......]
16 half shekel aa -reed, 1 shekel tamarisk seed, total: [19 drugs for ...].

. i

4 [............................] crushed [.........
5 [.............................] a n , tamarisk,
6 [................................]... coloquinth,
7 [................................], .adn -shrub, liquorice,
8 [...........................], "little-wine"-plant, "discharge"-stone (.),
9 [-stone], ib -sulphur, -sulphur, aaa -sulphur
10 [pappa -sulphur] aa , old cedar, cypress,
11 [.adn], a d , juniper, , ana , myrrh,
12 male and female [niip], n , human semen,
13 [pig-bristles], ox hoof, daina of the wash-basin,
14 [total:] 19 drugs as an ointment for fever.

The colophon identifies this text as part of the first tablet of the series Qutāru, dealing with fumigation (see Finkel 1991). Just as this manuscript was going to press, I discovered an additional source text for this medical commentary from Babylon (BM 44243), a Late Babylonian tablet in landscape format containing several clauses from the opening lines. A fuller edition of this text will be given later on, but the fact that a partial duplicate existed in Babylon shows that the source text was widely known.

Notes

1 Studies showed that in Crete people had high levels of fat in their diet combined with low levels of heart attack, but because the results from Crete were exceptional, they were generally ignored (see Agatston 2003: 16f.).

2 Beaulieu writes that "cuneiform writing was the preserve of a small caste of professionals" (Beaulieu 2007: 473). He supports his argument by citing a letter of 667 BC from a court astrologer addressed to King Esarhaddon, in which the astrologer twice quotes a popular proverb that "the scribal arts (*ṭupšarrūtu*) are not listened to in the marketplace" (SAA 8 338: 7 and 342: 7). The astrologer, however, is not making a general statement about literacy but was asking to have a private audience with the king; the proverb reinforces his point that academic subjects are to be discussed within the proper setting of the royal palace.

3 See, for instance, Walker 1990: 43: "literacy was not widespread in Mesopotamia. The scribes, like any craftsmen, had to undergo training, and having completed their training and become entitled to call themselves dubsar, 'scribe' they were members of a privileged elite who might look with contempt on their fellow citizens. Writing 'Ibni-Marduk dubsar' was the equivalent of writing George Smith, B. A."

4 See Healey 1990: 202f., referring to the alphabet as a "glorious simplification," although acknowledging the problem that the first alphabets made no allowances for vowels.

5 Von Weiher 1983: No. 22; von Weiher 1988: No. 85; see Fincke 1998: 29–31.

6 See Rochberg 2004: 257f.; e.g. in contrast to ancient omens, we assume today that the occurrence of thunder has nothing to reveal about the future of government.

7 Daryn Lehoux, (communication, Max Planck Institut für Wissenschaftsgeschichte, July 2, 2008).

8 According to the historian of Chinese medicine, Paul Unschuld, there is a distinction between "healing arts" (*Heilkunst*) and "medicine" (*Heilkunde*).

He points out that *Heilkunst* has no formal theoretical or scientific basis to explain disease or healing techniques, but is simply based on a tradition that disease emanates from gods or demons. *Heilkunde*, on the other hand, is based upon understanding disease as a function of laws of nature which can be explained without reference to divine causes (Unschuld 2003: 19ff., 55ff.).

9 French 2003: 18. There was much disagreement between Greek schools of thought in general about causes. The author of the Hippocratic treatise on *Ancient Medicine*, for instance, argued against the overly simplistic theory ascribing everything to powers of the four elements, earth, air, fire, and water.

10 We get some fresh perspectives on this close relationship between prognosis and omens by looking at Galen's experiences in his early years in Rome when he indulged in prognosis, which was not something Roman physicians were in the habit of doing. According to Roger French,

> The Hippocratic text on prognosis is not a reasoned argument but a description of signs that bode ill or well. This was uncomfortably close to the soothsayers' practice of seeking signs in entrails or the flights of birds, particularly since both practices were based on a knowledge of what was normal, in order to identify the abnormal. No doubt Galen remembered being called a soothsayer when he first made a prognostication in Rome. (French 2003: 51)

11 It is possible to imagine a rudimentary medical instrument such as a reed used to listen to the chest, but so far no medical instruments have been identified by archaeologists.

12 French 2003: 37, also pointing out that the Hippocratic treatise *Ancient Medicine* was a forerunner to a school of thought which took an Empiricist approach to medicine, preferring experience to logic and philosophy.

13 I am grateful to Gilles Buisson for the reading of Hammurabi's name in this tablet. There are several potential problems with this reading. First, Hammurabi is mentioned without his title "lugal," except that a similar reference to Hammurabi appears in another medical text from Assur, BAM 159 iv 22, in another recipe for eye disease: *te-qit* igi.min-*šú šá* ^{m}*Ha-am-mu-ra-bi lat-ku*, "a tested salve for Hammurabi's eyes"; see also BAM 382: 11, another New Babylonian tablet from Babylon with a salve for Hammurabi (*te-qit šá Ha-am-mu-ra-bi*). A third Late Babylonian Uruk tablet with eye-disease recipes has a similar line, "*tēqītu šá Ha-mu-ra-bi la-tík-tú*, a proven salve of Hammurabi." The second problem with our Hammurabi's mother tablet is the fact that Hammurabi is spelled with "pi" rather than "bi," although this is also not a decisive objection. According to Streck 1999: 659f., attested late Old Babylonian references to Hammurabi's name from Larsa spell the name with "pi" (e.g. *Ha-am-mu-um-ra-pi*).

14 See SAA 10 155, a letter addressed to Esarhaddon from his astrologer, telling the king that the tablet he is using is defective, and that he has acquired a tablet from Babylon dating back to Hammurabi, which is more complete.

15 The colophon has been discussed several times, see Elman 1975: 31; Rochberg 2004: 215.

16 *Apkallu* sages, who flourished before the Flood and had mastered all wisdom later lost to post-diluvian generations, were considered to be the precursors of exorcists, and *apkallu* became an honorific title for distinguished exorcists.

17 See Stol 1991–2: 59f., for the claim that "doctors were free to experiment." But Stol's support for this statement is based upon the "ditto" (ki.min) structure of Babylonian recipes, which implies that if one recipe does not work, one should try a second one instead. These alternative recipes, however, cannot be proven to be the result of experimentation or trial and error.

18 A similar ambiguity exists within Greco-Roman medicine. Galen, for instance, in his work on simples, complained that one of his predecessors had written about medicinal plants without testing their properties, and had not tested what previous scholars had written about plants.

19 Cf. CAD Š/437; see BAM 378 iii 3′–6′: "the stone's *šiknu* is like the *šiknu* of an oven," "the stone's *šiknu* is like the skin of a wild cat ..., the stone's *šiknu* is like a lion's hide."

20 See Lloyd 2007: 133, and also French 2003: 20f. French reminds us that *physis* can mean "nature" and Aristotle's use of the term refers to the "nature" of things. A *physicus* in Latin came to mean "natural philosopher" or "medical man," and later "doctor."

21 See Marti 2005: 1, a letter from Aqba-Ahum to the King of Mari which includes the following clause: *aš-šum* [*ša*]*-am-mi-im ša ek-ke-tim* [*ša*] *be-lí ú-wa-e-ra-an-ni* [*a-n*]*a* giš.kiri$_6$ *ša às-qú-di-im aš-pu-ur-ma* [*ša-a*]*m-mu-um šu-ú iš-te-en-ma* [...] *is-sú-hu-ni-iš-šu* [*ù a*]*-na ṣe-er be-li-ia* [*aṭ-ṭar-d*]*a-aš-šu*, "regarding the drug against *ekketum*-disease, which my Lord instructed me (to acquire), I sent (someone) to the garden of Asqudum; the drug was a *simplicium* and they dug it up and I have just sent it to my Lord." Marti translates the crucial phrase, "il y en avait une seule," but it is somewhat difficult to imagine that Asqudum's garden only had one variety of plant in it. Since *sammum* can also mean "drug," in this case the drug for *ekketum*-disease, it is likely that Aqba-Ahum wished to specify that he was sending this particular plant (or drug) because it was a *simplicium*, and hence other ingredients would not be necessary. A further intriguing question is whether the owner of the medicinal garden, Asqudum, was the well-known *bārû* haruspex in Mari (see Durand 1988: 593f.).

22 It is difficult to distinguish between plants used for drugs and plants used for ordinary culinary purposes or as herbs for seasoning, etc. (see Worthington 2003: 5–7). Texts dealing ostensibly with garden plants may actually have been used for medicinal purposes (see Röllig and Tsukimoto 1999: 427–39),

or for planting of herbs, although many of the same herbs appear in the medical corpus.

23 Maimonides in one of his treatises advises the patient (when no doctor is available) to resort to simple rather than complex remedies in the first instance, and if compound remedies are to be used, better one with fewer than many ingredients. Maimonides may have been repeating an older aphorism that one begins with simple recipes in preference to complex ones. In fact, lengthy Akkadian compound recipes may reflect academic medicine rather than actual prescriptions, which tended to be much shorter.

24 There is an unexplored connection with Babylonia here, since Erasistratos' father was court physician to Seleucus I.

25 Even Galen was unable to dissect human corpses but studied the bodies of apes (see von Staden 1998: 139f.).

26 Akkadian *libbu*, "heart," can also designate the stomach or internal organs of the abdomen in general.

27 See Heeßel 2004: 105–7, remarking that the usual principle of divination texts of distinguishing between "left" and "right" as partial determinants of good and bad portents is not valid for prognostic omens in the Diagnostic Handbook. This suggests that diagnoses and prognoses adhered more closely to actual observation than to theoretic principles of interpretation.

28 One might argue that collecting of symptoms from head to foot was intuitive, since Greeks collected them in a similar fashion, but the fact that no counterpart to diagnostic omens has been found in Egyptian medicine argues against this position.

29 For instance, the combinations of drugs in compound recipes may have reflected common knowledge about the effects of individual drugs, such as causing constipation or diarrhea, and hence known side-effects of a particular drug would have to be counteracted by another drug within the recipe.

30 One exception is BAM 7 34: 18–19, which reads: "if a man suffers from 'sun-fever,' flatulence, paralysis, lameness, *šaššaṭu*-disease, Hand of the Ghost(-disease), Hand of the Oath, disease of the rectum, (or) any disease: in order to cure him, …"

31 See the Hippocratic treatise *On the Sacred Disease* 21:

> A man with the knowledge of how to produce by regimen dryness and moisture, cold and heat in the human body, could cure this disease too provided he could distinguish the right moment for the application of what is beneficial, without recourse to purifications and magic. (Trans. Loeb; see Lloyd 2003: 71)

32 See Attinger 2008: 27 n. 37. The Nineveh manuscripts of these recipes have been edited in Cadelli 2000 (not in Attinger's bibliography).

33 See most recently Westenholz and Sigrist 2006; *muhhu* is otherwise translated as the "top of the head," which makes little sense in this anatomical

context. "Marrow" might serve as another meaning for *muhhu* appropriate to medical contexts.

34 Although not complete, tablets of this series have been edited by Attia and Buisson 2003 and by Worthington 2005 and 2007; see also Attinger 2008: 25 n. 34.

35 But see Geller 2007: 197f. for disease associated with this term, also in Greek.

36 Akkadian love charms from the third millennium show a completely different side to this literature, probably reflecting folk magic of the time (see Cunningham 1997: 58–60). This distinction between formal Sumerian magic and Akkadian folk magic will persist into much later periods.

37 See BRM 4 18, an incantation against the evil machinations of a witch for which no recent edition is available; see Abusch 2002 : 84 (also p. 12) for the opening lines: "she has fed me her no-good drugs, she has given me to drink her life-depriving potion, she has bathed me in her deadly dirty water, she has rubbed me with her destructive evil oil." The text then says (in Akkadian) that "Asalluhi saw him (the patient), he spoke to his father Ea: 'My father, as for mankind which (your) hands created, a witch has acted to reverse a man's breath …'."

38 There are other texts which, although not included in the series Maqlû, contained incantations with similar themes, see Abusch 2002: 89–92. In one such text (*LKA* 155), the patient refers to his terrifying dreams, pains in his neck and muscles, paralysis, impotence, and his being downcast, gloomy, and constantly crying.

39 See CAD B 219.

40 Some comparisons can be drawn between Greek *psyche*, which can also refer to the "mind" or intellect, and Akkadian *ṭēmu*, "reason, intelligence," since the Akkadian expression for mental illness is that the patient's "reason is altered" (*ṭēmu šanû*), or that his reason is confused.

41 See Stol 1999: 65. Similar texts can be found (in cuneiform copy) in BAM 228–32, but BAM 231 has been translated in Stol 1999: 66. Another example of this genre, *KAR* 26, was edited with duplicates and translated by Mayer 1999.

42 See col. ii 8–23 and Fincke 1998.

43 Although the first incantation is pseudo-Sumerian, the second incantation means "receive the prayer" (a-ra-zu šu-te-ma-ab).

44 See Appendix below, TCL 6 34 iii 3′–10′, a recipe for fumigation and a salve for "heartache" which includes various drugs (some exotic), which is yet another example of medical means to counteract a psychological disorder.

45 This is because the left is always "sinister" for the omen seeker but may indicate good fortune for his enemy or rival.

46 Babylonian doctors, like Greek colleagues, were warned against treating terminally ill patients, since death would reflect badly on the physician's reputation.

47 Koch 2005: 189, giving an earlier (Middle Assyrian) colophon from around 1100 BC which explains that the text was copied by the "chief of the diviners."

48 Caplice 1967: 41–4 reviews the use of terms for exorcist in Namburbî incantations, observing that although the logogram maš.maš or lú.maš.maš is commonly used, occasionally one finds a syllabic writing (*a-ši-pi*, Caplice 1967: 44), although the less common logogram lú.TU.TU is also encountered in these contexts, which we would suggest should be read lú.ku_4.ku_4, "the man who enters," alluding to the exorcist who enters the house of the patient to make a diagnosis, as known from the opening line of the Diagnostic Handbook.

49 Wiping is also one of the important ritual acts in Sumerian incantations, translated by the Akkadian *mašāšu* in bilingual contexts. We know "wiping" as *kuppuru* from Šurpu rituals, but *mašāšu* and *kapāru* are given as synonyms in a learned commentary; see for convenience CAD M/1 360.

50 One bilingual incantation begins, "I am the man of Nammu, I am the man of Nanše, I am the šim.mú, the 'plant-grower,' who heals the land, I am the great maš.maš who walks around in the city, I am the ka.pirig of Eridu who performs the mouth-washing" (Geller 2007: 106, 200). The Akkadian translation renders both šim-mú and ka.pirig as *āšipu*. Maš.maš gal.gal.la is translated as *mašmaš rabû*, the "great Mašmaššu-exorcist."

The fact that it was the exorcist and not physician who was expert in diagnostic and physiognomic omens is obvious from Esagil-kīn-apli's listing of the curriculum of the art of exorcism (*mašmaššūtu*), in which he lists the series *sakikkū* (the Diagnostic Handbook) as well as the physiognomic omen series *alamdimmû*, *nigdimdimmû*, and *kataduggû* as components of the training of an exorcist (*KAR* 44: 6; see Jean 2006: 64; see also Finkel 1988).

51 Like in earlier lexical lists, the exorcist is identified in the right-hand column of the lists as *a-ši-pu* in the sources (rather than *mašmaššu*), showing that *āšipu* was the preferred scholastic term for exorcist.

52 Rather than indicating that the diviner was an exorcist, this late reference probably alludes to the fact that the exorcist, in late periods, was the scholar who copied *bārûtu* divination texts. There was little scope for secular divination after the Persian period, since there was no Babylonian royal court.

53 See Parpola 1993: 327, with "exorcist" written with the logogram maš.maš (once lú.me.me in SAA 4 166). But exorcists in these letters practiced *a-ši-pu-tú* (SAA 10 352: 19); see SAA 10 160 and 275 for other syllabic spellings. Nevertheless, the title of Chief Exorcist (*rab āšipi*) is once spelled out syllabically as lú.gal *a-ši-pi* (SAA 4 316: 18).

54 Even the CAD article on *āšipu* (A/2 435) recognized that in one Namburbî text, *LKA* 108, the terms lú.maš.maš and lú.mu_7.mu_7 (Sumerian for "incantation priest") occur within the same context in successive lines and seem to refer to different persons. One lú.mu_7.mu_7 cracks a whip and recites an incantation and immediately afterwards a lú.maš.maš recites other incantations before the king.

55 One academic lexical list (MSL 14 223) associates Sumerian išib, a purification priest, with *āšipu* (not *mašmaššu*), *išippu, ramku*, and *pašīšu*, all various types of purification priests known from second millennium temple cults, (see Renger 1969: 122–6, 160–72).

56 *Pace* Kinnier Wilson 1972: 74, relying upon Landsberger's previous assumption that the *āšipu* was a scholar and man of letters but not priest. The assumption does not reckon with clear evidence of exorcists operating within the temple and receiving prebends, although one must allow for the possibility of lay exorcists as well.

57 See Jakob 2003: 529, citing an *āšip šarre*, royal exorcist.

58 See van Driel 2002: 36 n. 6, who states that "the gods did not need the *asû*, a mere medical practitioner," although he does not rule out any future discoveries of a medical prebend. As for the *āšipūtu*-prebend, see McEwan 1981: 71–3, although his reference (p. 73) to NCBT 1954 giving a *mašmaššūtu*-prebend is incorrect (collated); see also Bongenaar 1997: 288, giving evidence from Isin for a prebend for an exorcist, lú.zabar; and see also Seleucid prebend documents given by Corò 2005: 146–52, which refer to the exorcist's prebend by the more formal title *āšipūtu*, written out syllabically.

59 It used to be taken for granted that in the second millennium the *bārû* was a priest (see Renger 1969: 203–23). The assumption of the *bārû* being a priest is an easy one to make; like a priest, he performed rituals invoking gods when performing extispicy. The *bārû*, however, was more closely associated with the palace rather than with the temple, and his chief role was to advise kings on matters of state importance. This presumes that the *bārû* would have found animals for extispicy among the many banquets and meals served within the palace, rather than relying upon sacrificial animals used by the temple. The problem is that the *bārû* required numerous animals, over a long period of time, to create his *bārûtu* "database," from which he could derive the basic information he needed for predictions. If an event (to be interpreted as good or bad) happened on a certain day, associated with a particular shape of animal liver examined under special conditions, the database would provide crucial diagnostic information for the *bārû*: did this same peculiar liver shape ever occur previously, and, if so, what were the events at that time associated with it? The analogy would provide the *bārû* with a clue as to the interpretation of present circumstances, and whether events associated with the later extispicy were to be interpreted as favorable or unfavorable. See also Parpola 1983, with clear evidence from the seventh century BC for the *bārû* as a scholar, with similar interests to other scholars, such as exorcists and scribes.

60 The scribe was known as *ṭupšarru-Enūma-Anu-Enlil*, and McEwan 1981: 15 posits that astrology replaced extispicy in Hellenistic Babylonia. Another factor in the decline of the role of diviners may have been the shift in political power from Babylonia to Persia and the lack of a king for the *bārû* to advise.

61 See van Driel 2002: 115f.; Koch 2002: 140. We have one record of *bārû*-diviners in the Persian period who received temple rations (Jursa 2002: 112), and a *bārû*-diviner takes part in a building ritual in a text from Hellenistic Uruk (Linssen 2004: 103, 293/295: 22), although in neither case can the diviner be shown to be an active priest (references courtesy P.-A. Beaulieu).

62 Nevertheless, the Aramaic term *asya* may have lost its professional prestige; cf. Babylonian Talmud Kiddushin 4:14, which recommends not adopting low-grade professions such as a camel driver or physician.

63 The tale is The Poor Man of Nippur, for which see Foster 1993: 829ff. and now Dietrich 2009: 346f.

64 For an important case of an epidemic in Mari, see Attinger 2008: 45, citing Durand 1988: 17–20, in which the king is advised to stop in Terqa and not carry on to Saggarâtum, because of a widespread epidemic contaminating the region.

65 See Attinger 2008: 3, 50–1. The Code is often cited for the wrong reasons by historians of medicine, usually as an example of how cataract surgery was performed in Mesopotamia, or assuming the physician to be a type of priest (see Meyer-Steineg and Sudhoff 1927: 14). The value of the Code for medical history is limited, since the procedure described cannot be verified by evidence from the medical corpus itself. Nevertheless, the Code is one of the few documents from the period offering insight into the social context of medicine, and it shows that in the first quarter of the second millennium BC, the *asû*-physician was the only healing professional taken into consideration by the Code. The exorcist, on the other hand, did not have the same status or recognition and was probably seen as a priest (perhaps not even a designated priest) who recited incantations and performed rituals, but not in the professional capacity of being an exorcist. In other words, in this period, the priest was an exorcist, while in later periods the exorcist was a priest.

66 The Hittite legal code also tried to regulate the physician's income from patients, in a legal clause dealing with one man wounding his fellow of equal status. The man wounding his fellow must provide substitute labor to compensate for the injured man's inability to work (offering either a slave or himself), and afterwards, when the patient is healed, an additional sum of shekels must be paid in compensation, with 3 shekels of silver being given to the physician (Burde 1974: 2–3).

67 *muškēnu.*

68 *še-er-ha-nam*, referring to sinews, muscles, nerves, or virtually any soft tissue in the body.

69 Attinger 2008: 73 remarks that the *asû* is associated in early lexical texts with barbers (ED Lu E 47ff.).

70 A disease caused by breaking a taboo.

71 These letters have been studied in detail by J.-M. Durand and much of what we present here has been discussed previously in his seminal work on the archive.

72 See Durand's comments in Durand 1988: 555–7; Abrahami 2003: 19; and Attinger 2008: 44–5.

73 Finet 1957: 135 and Durand 2002: 306, referring to the lú.*a-si-im ša* é-*it te-er-tim*, "du médecins du bureau d'administration."

74 In Akkadian *šammu*. The word for "plant" in Babylonian can also mean "drug," and usually refers to what French calls a "simple," that is a drug consisting of a single (herbal) ingredient.

75 See Durand 1988: 552f. for a discussion of this ailment. Durand suggests comparing it to "Rose of Jericho" or "Bouton d'Orient" which are non-contagious skin ailments common in the Euphrates region. Durand concludes that *simmu* is likely to be a general term for any number of skin ailments, and it is not sensible to try to be more specific.

76 Durand 2002: 305 note d.

77 The condition known as *himiṭ ṣēti* is a type of fever associated with daylight or sunlight, difficult to identify in modern terms (see Stol 2007: 22–39).

78 *ṣītu*. See Durand 1988: 552, citing another letter (A.1494) in which *simmu* has broken out on a woman's neck, treated by a bandage; see also ibid. 578.

79 See Heimpel 2003: 279.

80 See Geller 2007b: 11, 60, describing a painful abscess, "its name is *ziqtu*."

81 Cf. incidentally another Mari letter (Durand 1988: No. 263; see Heimpel 2003: 279), reporting that the exorcist (*mašmaššu*) and lamentation priest (*kalû*) work together to purify a town or village, and as a result an angry god has become reconciled. We note the use of the term *mašmaššu* for "exorcist," although the term *wāšipu* is also known in Mari.

82 The majority are *pašīšu*-priests, with one *šandabakkum* (temple administrator), and one witness with the less grand titles of *rakbum* (messenger) and *kisalluhhum* (courtyard sweeper).

83 One of the house purchasers appears to be a *pašīšu*-priest of Šamaš, which may provide the connection with the temple.

84 See Schwemer 2007: 28 n. 24 for collations of the opening passage of this text.

85 *Dreckapotheke*, see below.

86 Infection caused by a dog-bite is described as a puppy being born under the victim's skin (Finkel 1999).

87 See Renger 1969: 143–72. It is difficult also to determine any precise etymological relationship between the terms išib/*išippu* and *āšipu*, although one suspects there is one. Cf. also al-Rawi and George 1994: 137: 7, a Neo-Babylonian letter mentioning a *pašīšu*-priest (in a later source than we would expect), but this letter turns out to be pseudepigraphic, purporting to be from Hammurabi's successor more than a millennium earlier. It is likely that by the first millennium the term *pašīšu* becomes a general term for "priest," without any specific function associated with his title.

88 *ša pa-na ma-a'-da i-né-'e-i-šu i-na-an-na ul i'-i'-iš*. The term used in this phrase for "feeling well" (*nêšu*) is the standard term used frequently in medical texts to describe the results of administering a recipe, *in'eš*, "(the patient) will get better."

89 *ša pa-na i-ge-en-ni-[hu] i-na-an-na [ul i-ge-en-ni-ih]*. The restoration is based upon the same phrase which occurs in another letter (Parpola 1983: 494, 13–14).

90 *šu-ul-mu ši-ir-ši-na ṭa-ab*, "their flesh is good."

91 *ihzu*, presumably referring to their training as singers and musicians.

92 *na-hu-ri-ta-ša iṭ-ṭi-ba-aš-ši*, "her *nuhurtu*-disease has got better," which may provide a clue as to the name of the disease. In any case, the discoloration appears to be a good sign.

93 Parpola 1983: 494. The first part of this proper name is damaged and our restoration of the name is provisional, based on the copy published in BE 17/1.

94 Bēlum-balāṭi may have tried to impress his boss (the king?) by blinding him with science and insisting that his recipes must include all available drugs.

95 Galen wrote a treatise of five books on simples, in which he defines simples by isolating their properties (e.g. emetics, causing sneezing or coughing, or having heating or cooling properties). He also composed a treatise on compounds in which he explains the side-effects of different drugs within a compound that had to be taken into account, as well as the combined effects of individual drugs being used together (courtesy John Wilkins).

96 I have been told that in India patients prefer compounds and hence physicians often prescribe a compound drug with only one active ingredient, to satisfy the expectations of the patient. The idea is that a good doctor possesses more complex recipes. Maimonides, on the other hand, preferred simples to compound recipes.

97 Resins of *nuhurtu* and *patrānu*, listed as plants used for abdominal cramps (*kīs libbi*); *merginānu, ararijānu, namruqqu, ulānu*, seed of "single"-plant, *kurkanû, hašânu*, among other plants.

98 Thanks to Maria Grazia Masetti-Rouault for showing me this text prior to publication.

99 A similar kind of complaint from a ruler is found in a prayer of the king Šamaš-šum-ukīn in a *šuilla*-prayer (Nergal 1), in which the king, in the first person, acknowledges himself to be "tired, wearied, and sleepless" (*anhu šūnuha šudlupu*), seized by a high fever (*ummu dannu*) and *li'bu*-disease, while "loss (of movement)" and "stiffness" (*hulqu munga*) have weakened his whole body, and a serious illness (*murṣu lemnu*) is permanently bound to him (see Loretz and Mayer 1978: Nos. 61 and 67; reference courtesy Joel Hunt).

100 Cf. Jursa 2002: 112, an exceptional tablet from the Esagil Temple in Babylon from the late Achaemenid period, listing *bārû*-diviners as recipients of rations, which does not necessarily show that diviners were priests but shows that they were on the temple payroll (reference courtesy P.-A. Beaulieu). Jursa argues that the sixth-century BC Esagil archive from Babylon preferred payment for cultic personnel through rations rather than prebends, and that diviners, singers, lamentation priests, and exorcists

were all paid rations on this basis (Jursa 2008: 38). Nevertheless, the sparse evidence for such payments to the *bārû*-diviner does not prove his status as priest or temple functionary, although the situation in Babylon may have differed from that of other temples and cities.

101 See also Jursa 2005: 100, other archival documents from this same man in Babylonia, showing that he was a man of property. He also owned an *ērib bīti* prebend, so was a priest, which makes sense in the context of SAA 10 160.

102 See Frame 1992: 131f. This letter is also discussed by Beaulieu 2007: 478. The suggestion that it may have been composed after the revolt of 652 BC raises further questions about when it was written. Hunger 1987: 162 assigns three possible dates to the letter, based upon astronomical data: June 672, 660, or 648 BC. Hunger opts for the middle date on the grounds that the letter was unlikely to be written from Babylonia after the revolt, but his assumption needs to be re-evaluated. The letter itself is in Babylonian script and must have originated in Babylonia.

103 But see SAA 16 65: 4–11, a letter from a goldsmith Parruṭu, who purchased a Babylonian for money (presumably a slave) and this Babylonian was entrusted with teaching Parruṭu's son various academic disciplines, including exorcism (*āšipūtu*), divination (*bārûtu*), and excerpts from celestial omens (reference courtesy E. Robson). This is the only instance I know of a slave acting as teacher.

104 Known as a *ṭupšarru Enūma Anu Enlil.*

105 We will see below that, within the scribal schools or academic system, scribes (or scholars) refer to themselves with the title tur (or bànda), "junior," and this qualification was only dropped when the scholar left school and operated within his profession.

106 See Falkenstein 1931a: No. 51, a ritual mentioning the *ilku* of the exorcist, lamentation priest, and singer, all temple personnel.

107 See Beaulieu 2007: 475, where it is stated that advanced students often learned a discipline from older family members. On the other hand, family relationships are not always to be taken as literal. For non-family members, the Hippocratic oath served as an oath of loyalty. See French 2003: 14f., explaining that the Hippocratic treatise on precepts was addressed to the writer's own group, expressed as "brothers" of a "family of physicians." The Hippocratic oath reflects, according to French, a "father-to-son type of education," in which the new recruit treats his teacher like a father.

108 Parpola 1987: 271n. 8 cites two other texts which appear to mention Urad-Gula, as physician and even Chief Physician (lú.gal.a.zu), but it seems highly unlikely for the same man to have held both these offices; we assume these to be different persons.

109 See Parpola 1987: 270, arguing that Urad-Gula was not actually reinstated after his father's letter to the king, and instead languished unemployed for several years, and as a result his petition is actually quite modest. Parpola's

analysis does not actually contradict our assumption that Urad-Gula was only able to write such a letter to the king because of a special relationship between exorcist and ruler.

110 Adad-šumu-uṣur's advice may have been based upon a hemerology listing lucky and unlucky days of the month, or it may have been based upon a specific calculation of when the Substitute King might be executed. A Substitute King was appointed after an eclipse or unfavorable omen considered to be dangerous to the reigning king, and the ritual provided for the king to step down from his throne for a period of time (of up to six months) in favor of his substitute, who was later executed, thereby fulfilling the ominous prediction. The Chief Exorcist, in this case, could have prohibited the princes from leaving the palace during the reign of the Substitute King.

111 We are not well informed about which category of scholars composed hemerologies. Exorcists may certainly have been candidates, since it is the *asû*-physician and not the exorcist who is usually prohibited in hemerologies from treating patients on specified days of the month.

112 SAA 10 316: 16: ^{ú}BU *^{ú}hat-ti*.

113 According to *The Guardian*, October 3, 2008, "Dan Ariely of Duke University [won a prize] for demonstrating that expensive placebos are better painkillers than cheaper ones." "Ariely's team told volunteers they were being given a new kind of painkiller, with some receiving an expensive one and others a much cheaper version. Even though all of them received the same sugar pills, those who thought their pills were more expensive reported less pain." There is no reason to believe that ancient patients were any less influenced by similar suggestions.

114 Although ^{šim}gig (*kanaktu*) does not appear in this tablet (AO 11447) probably belonging to Urad-Nanaya, this drug does appear in an Assur duplicate (BAM 3 iv 28), which contains closely related recipes for ear problems.

115 SAA 10 318: 8, Akkadian *unṭi* is translated as a "rash" (see Parpola 1983: 253), although the term is a variant of the term *hunṭu*, "fever," for which see Stol 2007: 21f. For another instance of free alternation of initial /h/ and /'/ in Neo-Assyrian, see Hämeen-Anttila 2000: 14, where the demonstrative pronoun *anniu* and *hanniu* can occur in the same text.

116 SAA 320: 11: *sa*-[*kik*]-*ku-šú* silim. Parpola's translation, "his pulse is sound" is attractive as a way of measuring the levels of temperature by taking the pulse, since an abnormally quick pulse is one way of determining high fever.

117 Following CAD Ṣ 187, translating *pariktu lipriku* as laying the bandages "crosswise," is to be preferred to the newer translation in CAD P 185, which follows SAA 10 315: reverse 12 and Parpola 1983: 237. The name *ṣilbu* may relate to West Semitic *ṣlb,* "cross."

118 *lu-šá-ah-ki-im*, (SAA 10 315: 13) which is a charged term, as we have seen above in Mari letters in which the approved medical expert is called *hākimu*.

119 Purging was commonly used in Hippocratic and later medieval medicine.

120 *ina* dúr-*šú ú-šeš-še-ram-ma iballuṭ*.

121 Cf. also Parpola 1983: 127; and for an edition of this ritual, see Tsukimoto 1985: 125–35.

122 Or "plant" (*šammu*), since the Akkadian term means both "plant" and "drug" (i.e. something which is not a plant extract); cf. Aramaic *sm'*, "drug" or even "poison," corresponding to Greek *pharmakon*.

123 It is often thought that the diviner was used to test the results of other types of prognostication, as a check to validate results, but in this particular case, it seems more likely that Adad-šumu-uṣur's trial would be more decisive, at least to determine if the drug was dangerous or had immediate side-effects.

124 The Diagnostic Handbook shows two general types of symptoms, those which recur regularly and supplementary symptoms which are uncommon but noteworthy.

125 The idea that disease has a "seat" within the body has parallels within Greek medicine.

126 Von Weiher 1983: No. 22, 120, and see also ll. 131–2, stipulating a fee of 7 grains of silver and 4 grains of gold for Šamaš, presumably to be paid to the *mašmaššu*.

127 A provincial eighth-century site in eastern Turkey.

128 The river god in the Sultantepe version probably serves as a metaphor for washing out the illness, comparable to the reference to rain in the eye in an incantation discussed above.

129 These medical incantations have relatively little in common with the great magical compositions such as Maqlû, Šurpu, and Utukkū Lemnūtu, which are much more complex and literary in both form and content.

130 Or has an erection.

131 Unlike his father, who held a position as exorcist in the Assur temple, Kiṣir-Nabû was an academic exorcist (*mašmaššu ṣehru*). His tablets were often excerpts for a specific reason, hastily made, probably for use within the scribal school curriculum (Hunger 1968: 20). Although he makes no claims to authorship of these tablets, it seems clear that excerpts for pedagogic purposes probably reflect his expertise as a scholar, with special interests in medicine and magic.

132 Cf. BAM 7 p. 210 colophon, where the sign *ana* should be deleted.

133 Presumably the consequences of violating an oath.

134 Suggesting that the recipe may have been very popular.

135 STT 97 iv 17–18 (not as noted in BAM 7 p. 174).

136 Another case of overlapping recipes occurs in a Nineveh tablet in Babylonian script (BAM 7 30). (N.B. tablets from the same period could be written in two different scripts, Assyrian or Babylonian, depending on whether they originate from Assyria in the north or Babylonian in the south; the script is not necessarily an indication of the dialect of Akkadian). Although most of this Babylonian-script manuscript is *not* duplicated in

other texts, two recipes are found in three other manuscripts from Assur and Nineveh, but in a different order.

137 It is difficult to assess the origins of Nineveh tablets in Babylonian script, but these may have been tablets brought to Nineveh from elsewhere to be copied by Assurbanipal's scribes for his library (see Parpola 1983b: 10f.). According to Galen, similar activities were carried out in the museum in Alexandria, where the rule was that any manuscript brought by ship to Alexandria had to be copied so that a copy could be deposited in the Alexandria library (see French 2003: 32).

138 BAM 19 and 20, and BAM 159 col. iv. One recipe also appears in a manuscript devoted to Hand of the Ghost-disease (BAM 165), indicated by symptoms affecting the bronchial tubes, eyes, and kidneys.

139 See BAM 7 plates 9 and 10. The tablet is numbered here according to the line numbering of the tablet itself as restored by duplicates.

140 Akkadian *kussû*.

141 See Böck 2008: 316 for a calculation that a single recipe contained 1,166 kg of plant-based drugs and 349.9 kg of mineral-based drugs.

142 See Böck 2008: 311f., showing that BAM 7 9 failed to note the parallel from BAM 430 for these lines.

143 Given by Böck 2008: 311: 13 as lul.tir-plant.

144 Reading šim.sal{.sal} (see Böck 2008: 314).

145 Böck 2008 emends this reading to *zi-bu-*⌜*ú*⌝.

146 See Böck 2008: 312: 24c (reading BAM 430 iii 3′); we would identify this plant with *alamû*, which is usually written with the logogram ^{ú}a.la.mú/ma$_4$.a.

147 Reading BAM 430 iii 36′ and 431 iii 39. Böck has correctly identified these duplicate lines.

148 The ingredients are commonly used in many different kinds of recipes and were probably readily available to any physician. This is one of a small group of similar tablets.

149 We referred to an earlier case of such experimentation at the Assyrian court, where a potion intended for the crown prince Assurbanipal was first given to servants, to test its effectiveness.

150 Empiricists, Dogmatists, Methodists, but these do not alter the general picture of the main characteristics of Hippocratic medicine.

151 See Harper 1997: 9ff., suggesting that Chinese medicine also developed an interest in nature after the third century BC. The Chinese did not develop natural philosophy along the same lines as the Greeks but nevertheless had their own observations of nature which they applied to medicine through analogy.

152 Dietary restrictions within Babylonian hemerologies, prohibiting certain foods on specific days of the month, were based upon magic and the notion of unlucky days, rather than upon maintaining a health regime.

153 Incantations occasionally considered prevention in the form of the incantation priest asking to be protected from the same demons who were attacking the victim, since demons were associated with the idea of contagion.

154 See Plato, *Charmides* 156d, reporting a conversation between a Thracian and Socrates: "as you ought not to attempt to cure the eyes without the head, or the head without the body, so neither ought you to attempt to cure the body without the soul." The Thracian adds that this "is the reason why the cure of many diseases is unknown to the physicians of Hellas" (Robinson 2006: 39).

155 Literally "grasp."

156 See Finkel 1988: 148f., in which Esagil-kīn-apli is said to have reworked texts which had been received as "'twisted threads' for which no duplicates were available."

157 In fact one of the main distinctions between court letters written to the king from exorcists and physicians is that exorcists consistently invoke the gods Nabû and Marduk in the opening address, while physicians invoke Ninurta and Gula. An exceptional royal court letter, SAA 10 297 (drawn to my attention by E. Robson), was jointly composed by the court physician Urad-Nanaya and the court exorcist Nabû-naṣir, reporting that the king's mother had recovered from her illness. Although this letter looks like an example of professional cooperation, the gods invoked are Ninurta and Gula rather than Nabû and Marduk, indicating that the letter actually emanates from the physician's secretariat, rather than that of the exorcist.

158 Although this particular tablet is partially duplicated in another Babylonian tablet from an unknown site, the final section of the composition is only known from Rīmūt-Anu's copy from Uruk (see Heeßel 2000: 353).

159 See Pedersén 1998: 206. A tablet of terrestrial omens (Šumma ālu) was copied by an exorcist (maš.maš) (see Falkenstein 1931: No. 128), as were Seleucid-period Uruk astronomical tablets belonging to exorcists (see Hunger 1968 Nos. 93–4).

160 See also Jursa 1999: 28f. for another reference to a Hellenistic archive of exorcists.

161 A contemporary archive from Uruk belonged to Iqīšâ, another *mašmaššu* with catholic tastes in reading, but some of his personal tablet collection may have been inherited from the earlier archives of Anu-ikṣur, since the two families of exorcists shared the same house in successive generations (see Pedersén 1998: 213; Robson 2008: 237).

162 The Akkadian loanword *magušu* seems to refer to a class of priests who took charge of temple affairs (CAD M/1 481f.), and we know that the *magušu* officiated in the Eanna temple in Uruk.

163 The status of the *mašmaššu* in Babylonian temples has little to do with the overall administration of the temples themselves under Achaemenid rule, since native Babylonians from important priestly families remained in

charge of the temples, with little evidence of Persians being appointed to such positions. For a useful overview see Fried 2004: 30f.

164 Written in esoteric orthography (common in colophons): lú [d]sin *u* [d]utu as a writing of lú *éš-u-tú* (= *asûtu*), "man of medicine." Urad-Nanaya was well known as Esarhaddon's chief physician, see SAA 10 254ff.

165 Such as the correct readings of logograms, e.g. the plant name NAM.TAR glossed in Akkadian as *pilû*, "mandrake" (see JMC 10 [2007] 11: 55).

166 Sumerograms hád.a sud, which the scribe glosses as *tú-ub-bal ta-sa-ka*, "you dry, you crush" (see JMC 10 [2007] 11: 59).

167 The term *šamallû* is a loanword from Sumerian (šagan-lá), although the original Sumerian term was purely commercial, referring to a merchant. The term can refer in late periods to a tradesman-like apprenticeship, such as a cook, or alternatively to a lamentation priest (CAD Š/1 294).

168 The term has no logogram despite being a loanword from Sumerian.

169 The family pedigree of a scribe was often considered worth mentioning in colophons. A few colophons (from Assur and Sultantepe) use a special word, *ligimû*, to indicate that the scribe is the "scion" of a certain family. For instance, the Sultantepe scribe who copied the literary text, *Ludlul Bēl Nēmeqi* (Poem of the Righteous Sufferer), refers to himself as an apprentice (*šamallû*) and "scion" of Ašû the priest (see Hunger 1968: 351 [= STT 33]). Another Sultantepe tablet (Hunger 1968: 360 [= STT 92]), a medical tablet assigning appropriate medicinal plants to various diseases, was signed by an apprentice (*šamallû*), "scion" (*ligimû*) and son of an Assyrian scribe. This term corresponds to another term popular among Assur scribes, *līpu* and *līp līpi*, "descendant."

170 See Rochberg 2004: 225, and Elman 1975: 20 for the similar *eširti ummâni*.

171 Reiner 1967: 199 tries to establish a hierarchy of scribal titles, as *agašgû*, *asû ṣehru*, *šamallû ṣehru*, based on this colophon of STT 301.

172 Hunger 1968: No. 318. See Lieberman 1990: 318f., in which he reviews the terminology in colophons claiming that Assurpanipal himself read the tablets – including *tāmartu*, "viewing," *šitassû*, "reading," *tahsistu*, "memorandum," and *tamrirtu*, "checking" – and argues that the reflexive /t/ forms of these verbs suggests Assurbanipal's personal involvement. Lieberman's argument is not convincing.

173 The tablet actually appears to be an excerpt from a hemerological compendium, but in any case a school text. Reiner 1967: 199 suggests that "reading" in this context could refer to checking the tablet.

174 See BAM 310, an etiquette which was probably attached to a group of medical tablets and has the label *maš-al-a-tú šá* sa.gig *mu-kal-lim-tú*, "questions and answers on *sakikkū* (diagnostic omens), a commentary." The etiquette ends with the label, "a tablet (lit. letter) of 27 aphrodisiac stones, lapis lazuli." See also George 1991: 152f.

175 Hunger 1968: 20. The two tablets in which Kiṣir-Nabû uses the phrase *ana malsûtišu* are BAM 52 and 106, although these belong to the same com-

position; see also BAM 147 for a similar Kiṣir-Nabû colophon, where *ana malsûtišu* might appear in the final damaged line. That this composition was copied from a wooden tablet from an Uruk original might be relevant, since the term *malsûtu* appears relatively frequently in Uruk texts.

176 See Hunger 1976: No. 12, and the one exception (No. 72), which is not listed as a commentary to extispicy but turns out to be a commentary after all (according to Hunger's notes on text No. 72).

177 The assumption is that *ṣehru* "junior" is not a diminutive in any sense, but is an exclusively academic title. Hence the difference between a *mašmaššu* and *mašmaššu ṣehru* is not "exorcist" and "junior exorcist" per se, but simply that a *mašmaššu* practiced his trade outside the academy, while the *mašmaššu ṣehru* was responsible for teaching exorcism within the scribal school.

178 The term *ummânu* would be the modern equivalent of calling one's teacher *Grossmeister*, which is a title only used honorifically or behind his back. However, some colophons come close to identifying the owner of a tablet as the *ummânu*, such as the following:

> *but-ṭu lat-ku šá* šu^{2} um.me.a dub ^{m}*ki-ṣir-*^{d}*aš-šur* maš.maš *aš-šur* (BAM 303: 24′–25′)
>
> tested recipe from the hands of the *ummânu*, a tablet of Kiṣir-Aššur, Assyrian exorcist.

Could Kiṣir-Aššur be the *ummânu*? It is difficult to tell, since a similar reference occurs in an eye-prescription text within the recipe itself: *te-qí-tu ša-lim-tu ša* šu um.me.a *la-ti-ik ba-r*[*i*], "a reliable eye-salve which has been tested and checked by the hand of the *ummânu*" (BAM 516 iv 4). The *ummânu* in this latter case is anonymous.

179 One argument in favor of this hypothesis is the number of colophons which mention the same scholar, in this case Anu-ikṣur, suggesting a certain level of popularity. Moreover, a reputable *ummânu* may have had the authority to edit and alter texts. E.g. one Anu-ikṣur tablet partially duplicates incantations for a crying baby known from Nineveh (Hunger 1976: No. 48, plate 143; Farber 1989: 60f.). This tablet, however, is unique in also presenting rituals against epilepsy and witchcraft, under the rubric of a standard series of medical recipes against fevers (Farber 1989: 21). It is possible that Anu-ikṣur himself was responsible for such an unusual arrangement of texts.

180 See George 1991: 152f., 162, translating one commentary colophon as, "commentary, oral explanation and question-and-answer dialogue according to a scholar."

181 Although not exact duplicates, each of the commentaries on the *Diagnostic Handbook* share similar traits and even explanations. Two commentaries, for instance, both quote from an omen text, Šumma ālu, to expound the same line of text (see George 1991: 155 n. 6). On the whole, the similarities

between commentaries can probably best be explained as oral traditions being passed down from earlier generations of scholars, although each centre of learning and each *ummânu* had his own unique method of expounding a text. It is this uniqueness which sets commentaries apart from other types of academic literature.

182 The common colophon phrase *ina pî ummâni*, "from the mouth of the Master," is a general expression implying that the knowledge is acquired through oral teaching; it does not purport to identify any particular *ummânu*, since the phrase is general and not specific.

183 George 1991: 152 gives the scribe's name as ^{md}*en-líl*-en-*šú-nu* ^{lú}maš.maš [tur$^{?}$] ⌜a-*šú* ^{m}*na*⌝-*ṣir* ^{lú}kul.lum ^{d}*en-líl* a ^{m}ab.sum.mu ⌜*šu-me-ru*$_{6}$⌝-*u*, "Enlil-bēlšunu's junior exorcist, son of Naṣir, divination priest of Enlil, descendant of Absummu the Sumerian." George suggests that the term "Sumerian" here may indicate that the scribe was from Nippur (George 1991: 160). The reading of the father's name is based upon badly damaged signs, and there is little evidence for the Sumerogram ^{lú}kul.lum to indicate "divination priest" (*bārû*). However, this same scribe appears again in Uruk, in a learned text, allowing us to correct the reading of the patronymic: ^{d}*en-líl*-en-*šú-nu* maš.maš.tur a *šá* ^{md}*en-lil*-zi-*tim*-šeš ^{lú}kul^{la}.lum$_{x}$(MUL) a ^{m}šu.^{d}30, "Enlil-bēlšunu, 'junior' exorcist, son of Enlil-napišta-uṣur, brewer," descendant of Gimil-Sīn. The esoteric writing ^{lú}kul.la.mul for ^{lú}kul.lum is based upon a convention that signs can occasionally be read backwards (i.e. /lum/ from /mul/). The meaning of this title is far from certain, despite lexical evidence relating it to Akkadian *sirāšu* "brewer," but this may be a pun on Akkadian *kullumu* "to reveal," which can refer to esoteric knowledge.

The ancestor given as "Absummu the Sumerian" occurs elsewhere in a Louvre tablet which may also come from Uruk, a scholarly explanatory text from the Persian period (reign of Artaxerxes) giving offerings associated with various groups of gods (Nougayrol 1947: 35, 28–32; Linssen 2004: 162 n. 277; see Hunger 1968: No. 123), and the author is given as "Zēr-kitti-lišir, son of Bēlšunu, 'junior' scribe, descendant of Ab-sum-mu the Sumerian." One wonders whether the name Bēlšunu in this colophon may be a hypocoristic writing of Enlil-bēlšunu, the same author of the Uruk commentary discussed above and descendant of Absummu the Sumerian. Furthermore, the name Zēr-kitti-lišir also appears in the patronymic of the scribe of the commentary (also probably from Uruk) which is edited below in the Appendix. All these scribes, Zēr-kitti-lišir, Enlil-bēlšunu, and Enlil-napišta-uṣur, may belong to various generations of the same family of scholars, and all of these scholars put their names to commentaries and explanatory texts, which may not be coincidental.

184 Although, as noted above, each commentary is unique, nevertheless there are some overlaps between the two Uruk commentaries which may indicate that the same scholar composed both tablets (see, e.g., George 1991: 146, 3 and 148, 22–3).

185 If *dannatu* is "stress," this would be the opposite of what the Diagnostic Handbook claims; it is obvious that the commentaries employ *dannatu* in another sense. See Finkel 2006: 141: 33–4, a commentary tablet which equates *dannatu* and *sunqu*, another word for "famine."

186 The Greek physician Diocles, roughly contemporary with Enlil-bēlšunu and Anu-ikṣur, taught that people who suffered from peripneumonia, "who are older than fourteen years, should be given little food" (see van der Eijk 2000: 169). It is true that no specific texts have ever been found from Babylonia which recommend diet and regimen for Babylonian patients, corresponding to numerous Greek texts offering advice on diet and fasting for patients; nevertheless, within the confines of the Babylonian school, we might expect some thought to be given to the medical uses of fasting.

187 This reference to the disease "dropsy" was also taken up by Anu-ikṣur, who remarks: "'dropsy' (means) not having a future"; (or) "'dropsy' (means that) one's future lacks good health" (George 1991: 148, 9b). This disease is considered to be either fatal or chronic and incurable.

188 Šumma ālu Tablet 49 (see George 1991: 146, 6a–b, 155). A commentary tablet from Borsippa on this very passage explains "captive woman" (*asirtu*) as a "concubine" (*esirtu*).

189 The Akkadian term *esēru*, "to confine" does not appear among technical terms used in medical texts, although the term *esēru* is attested in late Seleucid Akkadian, with the meaning of "confining a disease" (see CAD E 335). There may be an alternative explanation. The root *'sr* "to bind" is commonly used in Aramaic magic at the time this commentary was written, with its associated noun *asirta*, "(magically) bound (fem.)." Anu-ikṣur's interpretation of the passage may have relied upon a common Aramaic homonym, certainly known to Babylonians at that time, referring to a "bound" lilith-like demon entering the house.

190 Using the technical term *libbû*, "in this connection."

191 See Stol 2007: 11–15, giving evidence for *li'bu* mentioned in astronomical omens as being present throughout the country, and elsewhere being referred to as "*li'bu* of the mountain," probably indicating a widespread disease associated with a region. Stol does not consider *li'bu* to be a pandemic per se, but he does describe it as an infectious disease (ibid. 14).

192 *né-i-ir* sag.du *ma-hi-iṣ muh-hi* (Hunger 1976: No. 40, 6).

193 See Fincke 2000: 164, and similar expressions are attested describing the eyeballs as "grapes" or "raisins," probably all intending to describe bloodshot eyes.

194 See Leichty 1973: 83, with the variant that "the vine of the eyes is stretched so that the eyeball turns inward." This commentary was composed by Sīn-nādin-ahhê, otherwise unknown to me, and the provenance of the tablet is unknown.

195 Here we are forced to emend the text to *<na->ta-a-ka*; cf. Hunger 1976 No. 54: 16 bi.iz = *na-ta-ka*.

196 *niš-šú*, from *ni'šu* (see CAD N/2 283).

197 *ši-kin-ni*, either a form of *šikittu* or an error for *ši-kin-šú*!.

198 Restoring *pi-riš-tú* (?) from *JCS* 2 (1948) 307: 27. Whatever was stolen was probably taboo, and the ship may have been a cultic barge.

199 Another commentary on the Diagnostic Handbook takes a similarly pious view of things: "if a man is to recite a prayer, he will recover" (Dougherty 1933: No. 406, 14), which is a quote from the Diagnostic Handbook (Labat 1951: 88, 1).

200 Labat 1951: 36, 37 (dimin.bi), misunderstood by Labat as dkù-bi, and Hunger 1976: No. 30, 15, only citing the first part of the line.

201 Puns based on pseudo-logograms used to write the demon's name: šu-la-kù, with šu = "hand," la = "not," and kù = "clean."

202 Both the source text and commentary make the same mistake, using the word *šanānu* "to rival" for *šanû*, "to change" (both texts have *il-ta-na-an*) (see Labat 1951: 64, 58; Hunger 1976: Nos. 40, 7, and 41). The source text, however, is based upon a Nineveh manuscript, and we have no surviving Uruk manuscripts of this passage. It is conceivable that Anu-ikṣur worked from a Nineveh manuscript and copied the same error into his commentary.

203 The word *ensû* is given here as a homonym of *anšû* to rhyme with the bird.

204 *rikis murṣu naphar murṣu* (Hunger 1976: No. 39, 9). The idea of sa.gig = *riksu murṣu* also occurs in a commentary, *RA* 73 167 rev. 20 and in a lexical text (von Weiher 1983: No. 54, 13); the latter tablet belonged to Enlil-bēlšunu, the same *mašmaššu ṣehru* who composed the commentary on the Diagnostic Handbook discussed above (see also George 1991: 162; Finkel 1988: 148).

205 Cf. Labat 1951: 50, 12 which we can now restore from Hunger 1976: No. 31, 29f. as, diš igi.min-*šú ú-am-ma-aṣ* [úh-*šú* mur.meš šub.šub-*ma*] *ina* ka-*šú* du.[du], cf. AMT 105, 2. A parallel expression is found in another commentary, see Appendix below.

206 Another Uruk commentary (Hunger 1976: No. 41, 6) from the same milieu refers to a mishap befalling (lit. "seizing") a baby (based upon Labat 1951: 218, 9), which is explained as "Lamaštu-demon has chosen him." In the same way that the Maiden Lilith "chooses" her victims with sexual intent, the Lamaštu-demon "chooses" a baby as a victim; the same Akkadian word (*hiāru*) applies to both contexts. The commentary then elaborates on the baby being "behexed" (Labat 1951: 218, 19) by explaining that a "witch has driven him (the baby) to physical deficiency" (Akk. *maštaqtu*) (Hunger 1976: No. 41, 9).

207 Anu-ikṣur also comments on *pāšittu* in another of his commentaries, explaining this disease as "*pāšittu* (is) the Lamaštu(-demon) who 'strips' the body" (Hunger 1976: No. 49, 4). Anu-ikṣur may be alluding to the Aramaic root *pšṭ* meaning to "strip, flay, tear."

208 The Babylonian Talmud uses the idiom of "setting the table" to refer to having sex and "overturning the table" to having "unnatural" sex.

209 *i-ka-li-is-su*, interpreting this word transitively; the word is rare, but at least two attestations refer to the penis: "his penis is big but shriveled" (*kaliṣ*) (Clay 1923: 22: 28, cited CAD K 66) and the adjective *kalṣu*, also referring to a penis (CAD K 87, in a lexical context).

210 DAM-*su ul uq-tál-lal-ša*, not as interpreted by Böck or Hunger.

211 DAM-*su i-kan-nu-ša-aš-ša*, again not as interpreted by Böck or Hunger. A similar play on words is used in a second commentary on physiognomic omens (Hunger 1976: No. 84, 27), although this probably does not belong to Anu-ikṣur's work, but may have been a disciple or colleague, from the same Uruk archive. The text repeats the idea that "his wife will shrivel it" (using a synonym, the Akkadian word *ganāṣu*), but then adds that "she will run away from him." This second commentary fits very well with our interpretation of Anu-ikṣur's remarks on a similar passage.

212 Translation does not follow CAD T 300.

213 See Stol 1993: 11. The logogram an.ta.šub.ba is normally translated by the Akkadian word *miqtu*, "stroke," but another term for stroke or paralysis, *mišittu*, does not employ this logogram. The opening line of the commentary poses a difficulty, since it does not begin by quoting the incipit of the source text (TCL 6 34) but a line from the second column of this text, "(the term) 'stag's horn' (Sumerian) is translated by 'stag's horn' (Akkadian)." It is not clear why the commentary does this.

214 A similar comment was made by Anu-ikṣur based upon another passage from the Diagnostic Handbook.

215 *bēl ūri*, see Stol 1993: 16ff.; this particular disease-name appears to be synonymous with a more common term for epilepsy, *bennu*. The expression "lord of the roof" for epilepsy was borrowed into later Aramaic (cf. Kwasman 2007).

216 We encountered the condition *huṣṣi* above in another late commentary (Dougherty 1933: No. 406), and it is likely that both this and our commentary come from the same Uruk academy.

217 Hunger 1976: No. 49, 33–5. Anu-ikṣur also refers to the topos in another medical commentary (von Weiher 1988: No. 100, 12f.).

218 The connection with "owl's blood" may have something to do with the Sumerian logogram for "owl" (*qadû*), uru-hul-a^{mušen}, which literally means "bird in a bad city," perhaps alluding here to a leper colony.

219 See CAD N/2 222 and Riddle 1985: 132f. for a brief discussion of animal dung prescribed by Dioscorides.

220 There is also a medicinal plant known as "dog's tongue" (*lišān kalbi*), which was described as being useful for jaundice and cough, as well as against snakebite and dog-bite; the plant is so named, according to one ancient scholarly compendium, "because this is the plant upon which the geckoes lie" (CAD L 209).

221 The drying and moistening effects of drugs was a favorite theme of ancient and medieval medicine (see Edelstein 1967: 182f.). For Dioscorides and Galen on drug properties (including drying and moistening), see Riddle 1993: 105f., 115f.

222 For general explanations of how Babylonian commentaries worked, see Maul 1999 and Cavigneaux 1987.

223 There are recognizable similarities between commentaries ascribed to Anu-ikṣur and those later signed by Iqīšâ. See Robson 2008: 237f., explaining that the Šangû-Ninurta family (to which Anu-ikṣur belonged) had once inhabited the same house in Uruk which was later occupied by the Ekur-zakir family, of which Iqīšâ was a member. Although this does not prove any specific connection between the two scholars, it may suggest some continuity of roles within Uruk society.

224 There were resemblances between magic rituals and medical recipes, such as the use of fumigation in both magic and medicine; nevertheless magical rituals and medical prescriptions are still distinguishable by form and content.

225 E.g. dù.dù.bi = "its ritual," with "its" referring to the incantation.

226 Occasionally an alternative formula will be used: "In order to (treat a medical problem) ...". Medical literature from Babylonia always leaves the impression of being optimistic, in the sense that most medical remedies end with the positive statement that once the drugs are administered, the patient will get better or recover from his illness. Such statements are hardly realistic, since diagnostic texts, which list symptoms from many different types of diseases, often give a rather grim prognosis, that the patient will die or that the disease will persist for a time and then the patient will die.

227 For early second millennium (Old Babylonian period) texts, see Cavigneaux 1999: 253f., and for first millennium (Neo-Assyrian) examples, see Ebeling 1931.

228 The uses of these terms will be discussed below.

229 Similarly, in place of an abstract term for "divination," Akkadian uses *bārûtu*, the "art of the diviner" (*barû*), while "writing" is expressed by the term *ṭupšarrūtu*, the "art of the scribe" (*ṭupšarru*). There are abstract concepts in Akkadian, such as *nēmequ*, "wisdom," which is a form of *emqu*, "wise," or *ihzu*, "grasp," for knowledge or comprehension, but these are hardly abstractions in the Greek sense. There is also no actual Akkadian abstract term for "disease"; the word *murṣu* actually denotes "trouble" or "difficulty" but comes to be used specifically for illness.

230 See Parpola 1983: 8, discussing the fact that Nineveh library records from the reign of Assurbanipal in the seventh century BC provide data about private archives belonging to exorcists, diviners, and scribes, but each of the professional archives contains tablets from other disciplines, rather than from the specific area of professional expertise of the owner. It seems

clear that, by this period, specialists were more broadly trained in scholarship, beyond a single area of study.

231 See van Driel 2002: 113, referring to a text in which the temple barber has to inspect the bodies of priests as being suitable (unblemished) for priestly functions, including, theoretically, the king. This kind of inspection could suggest some degree of medical or physiognomic expertise.

232 Cf. TCL 6 34 ii 2; it is unclear why the commentary begins with a line from the second column of the source text, rather than with the incipit. The incipit of the source text appears in the second part of the opening line of the commentary.

233 Commentary based on TCL 6 34, 1–2 and duplicates: 1: [diš an.t]a.šub.ba ^{d}lugal.ùr.ra šu.dingir.ra šu.^{d}innin.na.

234 See Fincke 2000: 104–7.

235 Commentary on *ta-'a-šá hu-pat* sag.du *u* gú, "(you take) the *cover* of the cavities of the head and neck" (TCL 6 34, 4, duplicates AMT 35, 3: 3 and BAM 178: 2). See also [*š*]*u-up-lu* = *hur-ru* (depth = hole), Malku 2 62. The meaning of *šuplu* is not entirely clear in this context, although it may refer to the "pupil of the eyes" (*lamassatīnī*) of TCL 6 34 4, which occurs in this same phrase.

236 Cf. TCL 6 34, 5, ì hul ì ku$_{6}$.

237 TCL 6 34 iv 12.

238 múd buru$_{4}$.gi$_{6}^{mušen}$ (Akk. *āribu*), "raven-blood" occurs in TCL 6 34 iii 7.

239 See TCL 6 34, 6–7: kuš *an-dul$_{5}$-lim* ⸢*til-lat*⸣ *an-dul$_{5}$-lim*.

240 Cf. TCL 6 34, 2: máš^{zu} ti-*qé*.

241 In Akkadian *ruttītu*, a mineral, for which the Sumerian logogram is literally "river foam."

242 An unusual writing of the plant *šimmeššalû*, for which the conventional logogram is šim.šal, which we have later in this same line.

243 Cf. the Akkadian term *kukru*.

244 Logogram for both plants, *ballukku* or *nukkatu*, but since *ballukku* is represented in this line by another Sumerogram, šim.bulug, it is likely that *nukkatu* corresponds here to šim.mug.

245 e for è = Akkadian *waṣû*, come out.

246 A scholarly synonym for "plants" from lexical lists.

247 A writing of *buštītu*, "beetle."

248 Cf. the parallel passage, STT 93: 79–81 (cuneiform only), another scholarly text on the nature of plants (Šammu šikinšu) which quotes the same description of the *ašqulālu*-plant as in the present commentary but does not describe it as a "panacea," as in this commentary.

249 Cf. Geller 2007: 175, 214, in which *subandu* is the equivalent of the Sumerian ku.ku for "powder."

250 Copy has *a* for *ṣa*, emendation suggested in CAD S 309.

251 Copy has *ku*, emendation suggested in CAD A/2 302.

252 See Hunger 1968: No. 473, and see above.

253 Lines 4′–5′ of the reverse are characterized by having only a single oblique wedge used as *Glossenkeil* to separate entries in the commentary; it is not clear why the reverse differs from the obverse in this respect.
254 Derived from *uṣṣunu*, to cause something to reek?
255 = Akkadian *qaštu*; the bow of the ears, an unattested anatomical feature, although the Heb. term *qšt* is known, referring to a curved part of the stomach.
256 = Akkadian *ṣibûtu*, "need, require," "of what need there is."
257 A drug name.
258 Literally "bad-quality oil."
259 Based upon a.ri.a = *nawû* "steppe."
260 *Dreckapotheke*.
261 The entire phrase refers to a used sanitary towel.
262 There is a pun on "fox-flesh," since the Akkadian term *silqu* "beetroot" can also refer to "boiled meat."
263 *Dreckapotheke*.
264 A pun on another meaning of *šarūru* as a cucumber tendril; the meaning of "moon radiance" is more literary, and probably not appropriate here.
265 CAD G 50 has an alternative interpretation based on *kamû* as "captive," suggesting that a leper was incarcerated, which seems unlikely.
266 This comments on TCL 6 34, 6–7, in which "canopy hide" and "canopy tendril" are both *materia medica*.
267 The Akkadian term *edû* is usually glossed by the Sumerian /sig/ rather than /zu/, with a meaning of "recognized" or "prominent," which cannot refer to a goat. The point of the comment is that this type of goat is "well-known" in the sense of "commonplace" or familiar to everyone. Sum. zu is derived from the logogram máš.zu in a standard hermeneutical fashion.
268 *Dreckapotheke*.
269 Literally old cedar.
270 Variety or part of cedar.
271 See CAD B 352, citing this passage with the plausible explanation that the *buštītu*-beetle is associated with ^{giš}eren.sumun because the logogram for this beetle is gišhar, which consists of the signs /giš/ and /sumun/.
272 Based on the similarity of ù-mu-un and *amānu*, suggesting an etymological association between the words.
273 An expensive ritual anointing oil.
274 The homonym $bara_4$ is for bara, corresponding to Akkadian *halṣu*, "pressed," commonly used with oil, with an intended word play here between Sumerian bur "stone jar" and $bara_4$.
275 A drug for "every illness."
276 Possibly referring to the *allānkāniš*, the Kaniš oak, which can be chewed to assist in childbirth, but *allānu* is also a clyster.
277 Literally drug (for) forgetting grief.

278 Literally “locusts of the corner.”
279 *Dreckapotheke.*
280 A beer ingredient.
281 Tamarisk moss (lit. fungus) is associated with alum in Uruanna 3 50.
282 Interpreting the logogram literally, ú as *šammu* and ku_6 as *nūnu*. The term *kayyān* is the simple or literal meaning of a word (see George 1991: 155), rather than its second or third explanatory meaning, corresponding to the technical Rabbinic term *pešaṭ*.
283 The explanation is based upon a commentary on terrestrial omens (Šumma ālu) (see CAD A/2 302) and appears to be an unflattering equation between field pests and foreigners.
284 CAD T 300 reads [*ina*] *ši-lip* gír igi-*i*, “when the dagger is first(?) pulled out(?),” which is not convincing; we prefer the older reading in CAD L 60.
285 Cf. BAM 445: 26.
286 Restored from BAM 388 i 12.
287 Restored after BAM 179.

References

Abrahami, P. 2003. "A propos des fonctions de l'*asû* et de l'*āšipu*: la conception de l'auteur de l'hymne sumérien dédié à Ninisina," *JMC* 3: 19–20.

Abusch, T. 2002. *Mesopotamian Witchcraft* (Leiden).

Agatston, A. 2003. *The South Beach Diet* (London).

Algaze, G. 2008. *Ancient Mesopotamia at the Dawn of Civilization: The Evolution of an Urban Landscape* (Chicago).

Attia, A., and Buisson, G. 2003. "Edition de texte 'Si le crâne d'un homme contient de la chaleur, deuxième tablette'," *JMC* 1: 1–24.

Attinger, P. 2008. "La médecine mésopotamienne," *JMC* 11–12: 1–96.

Avalos, H. 1998. *Illness and Health Care in the Ancient Near East: The Role of the Temple in Greece, Mesopotamia, and Israel* (Atlanta).

Barton, T. 1994. *Ancient Astronomy* (London).

Beaulieu, P.-A. 2006. "Official and Vernacular Languages: The Shifting Sands of Imperial and Cultural Identities in First-Millennium BC Mesopotamia," in *Margins of Writing, Origins of Cultures*, ed. S. L. Sanders (Chicago), 187–216.

Beaulieu, P.-A. 2007. "Late Babylonian Intellectual Life," in *The Babylonian World*, ed. G. Leick (London).

Bernstein, A. E. 1993. *The Formation of Hell* (London).

Biggs, R. D. 1968. "An Esoteric Babylonian Commentary," *RA* 62: 52–7.

Black, J., Cunningham, G., Robson, E., and Zólyomi, G. 2006. *The Literature of Ancient Sumer* (Oxford).

Böck, B. 2000. *Die babylonisch-assyrische Morphoskopie* (Vienna).

Böck, B. 2007. *Das Handbuch* Muššu'u *"Einreibung"* (Madrid).

Böck, B. 2008. "Babylonisch-assyrische Medizin in Texten und Untersuchungen: Erkrankungen des uro-genitalen Traktes, des Enddarmes und des Anus," *WZKM* 98: 295–346.

Bongenaar, A. C. V. M. 1997. *The Neo-Babylonian Ebabbar Temple at Sippar: Its Administration and its Prosopography* (Leiden).

Briant, P. 2002. *From Cyrus to Alexander: A History of the Persian Empire* (Winona Lake).

Burde, C. 1974. *Hethitische medizinische Texte* (Wiesbaden).

Burkert, W. 2004. *Babylon, Memphis, Persepolis: Eastern Contexts of Greek Culture* (Cambridge, MA).

Cadelli, D. S. 2000. *Recherche sur la médecine mésopotamienne* (Paris/Geneva, unpublished PhD dissertation).

Campbell Thompson, R. 1924. "A Babylonian Explanatory Text," *JRAS*, 452–7.

Caplice, R. I. 1967. "Participants in the Namburbi Rituals," *CBQ* 29: 40–46.

Cavigneaux, A. 1981. *Textes scolaires du temple de Nabû ša Harê* (Baghdad).

Cavigneaux, A. 1987. "Aux sources du Midrash: l'hermeneutique babylonienne," *AuOr* 5: 243–55.

Cavigneaux, A. 1999. "A Scholar's Library in Meturan?" in *Mesopotamian Magic: Textual, Historical, and Interpretative Perspectives*, ed. T. Abusch and K. van der Toorn (Groningen), 251–73.

Charpin, D. 2004. "Lire et écrire en Mésopotamie: une affaire de specialistes?" *Académie des Inscriptions et Belles-Lettres*, Comptes Rendus (Paris).

Civil, M. 1960. "Prescriptions médicales sumériennes, *RA* 54: 57–72.

Civil, M. 1974. "Medical Commentaries from Nippur," *JNES* 33: 329–38.

Clay, A. T. 1923. *Babylonian Records in the Library of J. Pierpont Morgan* (New Haven).

Collins, T. J. 1999. *Natural Illness in Babylonian Medical Incantations* (University of Chicago, unpublished PhD dissertation).

Collon, D. 1987. *First Impressions, Cylinder Seals in the Ancient Near East* (London).

Corò, P. 2005. *Prebende templari in età seleucide* (Padua).

Cryer, F. H. 1994. *Divination in Ancient Israel and its Near Eastern Environment* (Sheffield).

Cunningham, G. 1997. *Deliver Me from Evil* (Rome).

Damerow, P. 2007. "The Material Culture of Calculation," in *Mathematisation and Demathematisation*, ed. U. Gellert and E. Jablonka (Rotterdam).

Dietrich, M. 2009. "'Armer Mann von Nippur': ein Werk der Krisenliterature des 8. Jh. v. Chr.," in *Of God(s), Trees, Kings, and Scholars: Neo-Assyrian and Related Studies in Honour of Simo Parpola*, ed. M. Luukko, S. Svärd, R. Mattila (Helsinki), 333–52.

Dougherty, R. P. 1933. *Archives from Erech, Neo-Babylonian and Persian Periods*, Goucher College Cuneiform Inscriptions 2 (New Haven).

Durand, J.-M. 1988. *Archives Epistolaires de Mari* 1/1 (ARM 26/1) (Paris).

Durand, J.-M. 2002. *Les documents épistolaires du palais de Mari* (Paris).

Ebeling, E. 1931. "Aus dem Tagewerk eines assyrischen Zauberpriesters," *MAOG* 5/3 (Leipzig).

Edelstein, L. 1967. *Ancient Medicine, Select Papers of Ludwig Edelstein*, ed. O. Temkin and C. L. Temkin (Baltimore).

Elman, Y. 1975. "Authorative Oral Traditions in Neo-Assyrian Scribal Circles," *JANES* 7: 19–32.

Fales, F. M. 2001. *L'impero assiro* (Rome).

Falkenstein, A. 1931. *Die Haupttypen der sumerischen Beschwörung* (Leipzig).

Falkenstein, A. 1931a. *Literarische Keilschrifttexte aus Uruk* (Berlin).

Farber, W. 1973. "*ina* kuš.dù.dù(.bi) = *ina maški tašappi*", *ZA* 63: 59–68.

Farber, W. 1977. *Beschwörungsrituale an Ištar und Dumuzi* (Wiesbaden).

Farber, W. 1989. *Schlaf Kindchen Schlaf! Mesopotamische Baby-beschwörungen und-Rituale* (Winona Lake).

Farber, W. 1989a. "Ki-sikil-u$_4$-da-kar-ra," in *Dumu-E$_2$-Dub-ba-a, Studies in Honor of Aka Sjöberg*, ed. H. Behrens, D. Loding, and M. T. Roth, 149–53.

Farber, W. 1999. "Dr. med. Apil-ilišu, Mārat-Anim-Strasse (am Ebabbar-Tempel) Larsa," in *Minuscula Mesopotamica: Festschrift für Johannes Renger*, ed. B. Böck, E. Cancik-Kirschbaum, and T. Richter (Münster), 135–49.

Farber, W. 2004. "How to Marry a Disease: Epidemics, Contagion, and a Magic Ritual against the 'Hand of a Ghost'," in *Magic and Rationality in Ancient Near Eastern and Graeco-Roman Medicine*, ed. H. J. Horstmanshoff and M. Stol (Leiden).

Fincke, J. 1998. "SpTU III Nr. 85 joint zu SpTU No. 22," *Nouvelles assyriologiques brèves et utilitaires* No. 26, 29–31.

Fincke, J. 2000. *Augenleiden nach keilschriftlichen Quellen, Untersuchungen zur altorientalischen Medizin* (Würzburg).

Fincke, J. 2006–7. "Omina, die 'Göttlichen Gezetze' der Divination," *JEOL* 40: 131–47.

Finet, A. 1957. "Les médecins au Royaume de Mari," *AIPHOS* 14 (1954–7): 123–44.

Finkel, I. L. 1988. "Adad-apla-iddina, Esagil-kin-apli, and the Series SA.GIG," in *A Scientific Humanist: Studies in Memory of Abraham Sachs*, ed. E. Leichty, J. Ellis, P. Gerardi, M. de J. Ellis, and O. Gingerich (Philadelphia), 143–59.

Finkel, I. L. 1991. "Muššu'u, Qutaru, and the Scribe Tanittu-Bel," Fs. Civil, 91–112.

Finkel, I. L. 1999. "On Some Dog, Snake and Scorpion Incantations," in *Mesopotamian Magic: Textual, Historical, and Interpretative Perspectives*, ed. T. Abusch and K. van der Toorn (Groningen), 211–250.

Finkel, I. L. 2000. "On Late Babylonian Medical Training," in *Wisdom, Gods and Literature: Studies in Assyriology in Honour of W. G. Lambert*, ed. A. R. George and I. L. Finkel (Winona Lake), 137–223.

Finkel, I. L. 2006. "On an Izbu VII Commentary," in *If a Man Builds a Joyful House*, ed. A. K. Guinan, M. de J. Ellis, A. J. Ferrara, et al. (Leiden), 139–48.

Foster, B. 1993. *Before the Muses* (Bethesda).

Foster, B. 2007. *Akkadian Literature of the Late Period* (Münster).

Frahm, E. 1999. "Nabû-zuqup-kēnu, das Gilgameš-epos und der Tod Sargons II," *JCS* 51: 73–90.

Frame, G. 1992. *Babylonia 689–627 BC: A Political History* (Istanbul).

French, R. 2003. *Medicine before Science* (Cambridge).

Friberg, J. 2007. *Amazing Traces of a Babylonian Origin in Greek Mathematics* (Singapore).

Fried, L. S. 2004. *The Priest and the Great King* (Winona Lake).

Geller, M. J. 2000. "Fragments of Magic, Medicine, and Mythology from Nimrud," *BSOAS* 63: 331–9.

Geller, M. J. 2003. "Mesopotamian Love Magic: Discourse or Intercourse?" *CRRAI* 47/1, ed. S. Parpola and R. Whiting (Helsinki), 129–39.

Geller, M. J. 2004. "Akkadian Evil Eye Incantations from Assur," *ZA* 94: 52–8.

Geller, M. J. 2004a. "West Meets East: Early Greek and Babylonian Diagnosis," in *Magic and Rationality in Ancient Near Eastern and Graeco-Roman Medicine,* ed. H. J. Horstmanshoff and M. Stol (Leiden), 11–61.

Geller, M. J. 2005. *Renal and Rectal Disease*, Babylonisch-assyrische Medizin in Texten und Untersuchungen VII (Berlin).

Geller, M. J. 2006. "Les maladies et leurs causes, selon un texte médical paléobabylonien," *JMC* 8: 7–12.

Geller, M. J. 2007. "Phlegm and Breath," in *Disease in Babylonia*, I. L. Finkel and M. J. Geller (Leiden), 187–99.

Geller, M. J. 2007a. "Incantations within Medical Texts," in *The Babylonian World*, ed. G. Leick (Abingdon), 389–99.

Geller, M. J. 2007b. "Textes médicaux du Louvre nouvelle édition," *JMC* 10: 4–8.

Geller, M. J. 2007c. *Evil Demons, Canonical Utukkū Lemnūtu Incantations* (Helsinki).

George, A. R. 1991. "Babylonian Texts from the Folios of Sidney Smith. Part Two: Prognostic and Diagnostic Omens, Tablet I," *RA* 85: 137–63.

George, A. R. 1993. "Ninurta-Pāqidāt's Dog Bite, and Notes on Other Comic Tales," *Iraq* 55: 63–75

George, A. R. 2008. "Review of Koch, *Secrets of Extiscipy*," *BSOAS* 71: 557–8.

George, C. 2002. "Development of the Idea of Chronic Renal Failure," *American Journal of Nephrology* 22: 231–9.

Gesche, P. 2001. *Schulunterricht in Babylonien im ersten Jahrtausend v. Chr.* (Münster).

Glassner, J.-J. 2007. "Lignées de lettrés en Mésopotamie," in *Lieux de Savoir, espaces et communautés*, ed. C. Jacob (Fondation des Treilles), 134–56.

Goltz, D. 1974. *Studien zur altorientalischen und griechischen Heilkunde, Therapie – Arzneibereitung – Rezeptstruktur* (Wiesbaden).

Gundert, B. 2006. "Soma and Psyche in Hippocratic Medicine," in *Psyche and Soma*, ed. J. P. Wright and P. Potter (Oxford), 13–35.

Hämeen-Anttila, J. 2000. *A Sketch of Neo-Assyrian Grammar* (Helsinki).

Harper, D. J. 1997. *Early Chinese Medical Literature: The Mawangdui Medical Manuscripts* (London).

Healey, J. F. 1990. "The Early Alphabet," in J. T. Hooker, *Reading the Past* (London), 197–257.

Heeßel, N. 2000. *Babylonisch-assyrische Diagnostik* (Münster).
Heeßel, N. 2004. "Diagnosis, Divination and Disease: Towards an Understanding of the *Rationale* Behind the Babylonian Diagnostic Handbook," in *Magic and Rationality in Ancient Near Eastern and Graeco-Roman Medicine,* ed. H. J. Horstmanshoff and M. Stol (Leiden), 97–116.
Heeßel, N., and al-Rawi, F. 2003. "Tablets from the Sippar Library XII: A Medical Therapeutic Text," *Iraq* 65: 221–39.
Heimpel, W. 2003. *Letters to the King of Mari* (Winona Lake).
Herrero, P. 1984. *La thérapeutique mésopotamienne* (Paris).
Hunger, H. 1968. *Babylonische und assyrische Kolophone* (= *BAK*) (Neukirchen-Vluyn).
Hunger, H. 1976. *Spätbabylonische Texte aus Uruk, Teil I* (Berlin).
Hunger, H. 1987. "Empfelhlungen an den König," in *Language, Literature, and History: Philological and Historical Studies Presented to Erica Reiner*, ed. R. Rochberg-Halton (New Haven), 157–66.
Jakob, S. 2003. *Mittelassyrische Verwaltung und Socialstruktur, Untersuchungen* (Leiden).
Jean, C. 2006. *La magie néo-assyrienne en contexte* (Helsinki).
Jeyes, U. 1980. "The Act of Extispicy in Ancient Mesopotamia: an Outline," *Assyriological Miscellanies*, ed. B. Alster (Copenhagen).
Joanna, J. 1999. *Hippocrates* (Baltimore).
Jursa, M. 1999. *Das Archiv des Bēl-Rēmanni* (Istanbul).
Jursa, M. 2002. "Florilegium babyloniacum: Neue Texte aus hellenistischer und spätachämenidischer Zeit," in *Mining the Archives*, ed. C. Wunsch (Dresden), 107–30.
Jursa, M. 2005. *Neo-Babylonian Legal and Administrative Documents: Typology, Contents and Archives* (Münster).
Jursa, M. 2008. "The Remuneration of Institutional Labourers in an Urban Context in Babylonia in the First Millennium BC," in *L'archive des fortifications de Persépolis*, ed. P. Briant, W. Henkelman, M. Stolper (Paris), 387–427.
Kinnier Wilson, J. V. 1972. *The Nimrud Wine Lists* (London).
Kinnier Wilson, J. V., and Reynolds, E. H. 2007. "On Stroke and Facial Palsy in Babylonian Texts," in *Disease in Babylonia*, ed. I. L. Finkel and M. J. Geller (Leiden).
Koch, U. S. 2005. *Secrets of Extispicy* (Münster).
Koch-Westenholz, U. 2002. "Old Babylonian Extispicy Reports," in *Mining the Archives*, ed. C. Wunsch (Dresden), 131–45.
Köcher, F. 1995. "Ein Text medizinischen Inhalts aus dem neubabylonischen Grab," in *Uruk – die Gräber*, ed. R. M. Boehmer, F. Pedde, and B. Salje (Mainz), 203–17.
Krispijn, T. J. H. 2008. "Music and Healing for Someone Far Away from Home: HS 1556, a Remarkable Ur III Incantation, Revisited," in *Studies in Ancient Near Eastern World View and Society* (Fs. Stol), ed. R. J. van der Spek (Bethesda), 173–93.

Kwasman, T. 2007. "The Demon of the Roof," in *Disease in Babylonia*, ed. I. L. Finkel and M. J. Geller (Leiden).
Labat, R. 1939. *Hémérologies et ménologies d'Assur* (Paris).
Labat, R. 1951. *Traité akkadien de diagnostics et pronostics médicaux* (Leiden).
Lambert, W. G. 1965. "Nebuchadnezzar King of Justice," *Iraq* 27: 1–11.
Lambert, W. G. 1967. *Babylonian Wisdom Literature* (Oxford).
Lambert, W. G. 1967a. "The Gula Hymn of Bulluṭsu-rabi," *Or* 36: 105–32.
Lambert, W. G. 1974. "*Dingir.šà.dib.ba* Incantations," *JNES* 33: 267–322.
Lambert, W. G. 1998. "The Qualifications of Babylonian Diviners," in *Festschrift für Rykele Borger zu seinem 65. Geburtstag am 24 Mai 1994*, ed. S. M. Maul (Groningen).
Leichty, E. 1973. "Two Late Commentaries," *AfO* 24: 78–86.
Lieberman, S. J. 1990. "Canonical and Official Cuneiform Texts: Towards an Understanding of Assurbanipal's Personal Tablet Collection," in *Lingering Over Words*, ed. T. Abusch, J. Huehnergard, and P. Steinkeller (Atlanta), 305–36.
Linssen, M. J. H. 2004. *The Cults of Uruk and Babylon: The Temple Ritual Texts as Evidence for Hellenistic Cult and Practice* (Leiden).
Livingstone, A. 1986. *Mystical and Mythological Explanatory Works of Assyrian and Babylonian Scholars* (Oxford).
Lloyd, G. E. R. 1979. *Magic, Reason and Experience: Studies in the Origin and Development of Greek Science* (Cambridge).
Lloyd, G. E. R. 1983. *Hippocratic Writings* (Penguin).
Lloyd, G. E. R. 2003. *In the Grip of Disease: Studies in Greek Imagination* (Oxford).
Lloyd, G. E. R. 2007. *Cognitive Variations* (Oxford).
Loretz, O., and Mayer, W. R. 1978. *Šu-ila Gebete, Supplement zu L. W. King, Babylonian Magic and Sorcery* (Alter Orient and Altes Testament 34, Kevelaer-Neukirchen-Vluyn).
Lucas, C. J. 1979. "The Scribal Tablet-House in Ancient Mesopotamia," *History of Education Quarterly* 19: 305–32.
Marti, L. 2005. "Recherche d'un remède contre le mal-ekkêtum," *JMC* 5: 1–3.
Maul, S. 1994. *Zukunftsbewältigung, eine Untersuchung altorientalischen Denkens anhand der babylonisch-assyrischen Löserituale (Namburbi)* (Mainz).
Maul, S. 1999. "Das Worte im Worte. Orthographie und Etymologie als hermeneutische Verfahren babylonischer Gelehrter," in *Kommentare*, ed. G. Most (Groningen).
Maul, S. 2004. "Die 'Lösung vom Bann': Überlegungen zu altorientalischen Konzeptionen von Krankheit und Heilkunst," in *Magic and Rationality in Ancient Near Eastern and Graeco-Roman Medicine*, ed. H. J. Horstmanshoff and M. Stol (Leiden), 78–95.
Mayer, W. 1999. "Das Ritual *KAR* 26 mit dem Gebet 'Marduk 24,'" *Or* NS 68: 145–63.

McEwan, G. J. P. 1981. *Priest and Temple in Hellenistic Babylonia* (Wiesbaden).

Meyer-Steineg, T., and Sudhoff, K. 1927. *Geschichte der Medizin* (Jena).

Milano, L. 2004. "Food and Identity in Mesopotamia: A New Look at the Aluzinnu's Recipes," in *Food and Identity in the Ancient World*, ed. C. Grottanelli and L. Milano, 243–56.

Neugebauer, O. 1955. *Astronomical Cuneiform Texts* (London).

Nougayrol, J. 1947. "Textes et documents figurés," *RA* 41: 23–53.

Nunn, J. F. 1996. *Ancient Egyptian Medicine* (Norman, Oklahoma).

Nutton, V. 2004. *Ancient Medicine* (London).

Oppenheim, A. L. 1943. "Akkadian *pul(u)h(t)u* and *melammu*," *Journal of the American Oriental Society* 63: 31–4.

Oppenheim, A. L. 1977. *Ancient Mesopotamia, Portrait of a Dead Civilization* (Chicago).

Parpola, S. 1983. *Letters from Assyrian Scholars to the Kings Esarhaddon and Assurbanipal. Part II: Commentary and Appendices* (Neukirchen-Vluyn).

Parpola, S. 1983b. "Assyrian Library Records," *JNES* 42: 1–28.

Parpola, S. 1987. "The Forlorn Scholar," in *Language, Literature, and History: Philological and Historical Studies Presented to Erica Reiner*, ed. R. Rochberg-Halton (New Haven), 257–78.

Parpola, S. 1993. *Letters from Assyrian and Babylonian Scholars* (= SAA 10) (Helsinki).

Pedersén, O. 1986. *Archives and Libraries in the City of Assur*, II (Uppsala).

Pedersén, O. 1998. *Archives and Libraries in the Ancient Near East* (Bethesda).

Porter, R. 1997. *The Greatest Benefit to Mankind* (London).

Radner, K. 2009. "The Assyrian King and his Scholars: The Syro-Anatolian and the Egyptian Schools," in *Of God(s), Trees, Kings, and Scholars: Neo-Assyrian and Related Studies in Honour of Simo Parpola*, ed. M. Luukko, S. Svärd, R. Mattila (Helsinki), 221–38.

al-Rawi, F., and George, A. 1994. "Tablets from the Sippar Library III. Two Royal Counterfeits," *Iraq* 56: 135–48.

Reiner, E. 1967. "Another Volume of Sultantepe Tablets," *JNES* 26: 177–200.

Reiner, E. 1995. *Astral Magic in Babylonia* (Philadelphia).

Renger, J. 1969. "Priestertum der altbabylonischen Zeit," *ZA* 59: 104–230.

Renn, J., and Damerow, P. 2007. "Mentale Modelle als kognitive Instrumente der Transformation von technischem Wissen," in *Übersetzung und Transformation*, ed. H. Böhme, C. Rapp, and W. Rösler (Berlin).

Riddle, J. M. 1985. *Dioscorides on Pharmacy and Medicine* (Austin).

Riddle, J. M. 1993. "High Medicine and Low Medicine in the Roman Empire," in *Rise and Decline of the Roman World*, Aufstieg und Niedergang der römischen Welt 37.1, Teil II Principat, ed. W. Haase (Berlin).

Ritter, E. 1965. "Magical-Expert (= *āšipu*) and Physician (= *asû*): Notes on Two Complementary Professions in Babylonian Medicine," in *Studies in Honor of Benno Landsberger on his Seventy-fifth Birthday April 21, 1965*, Assyriological Studies No. 16 (Chicago), 299–321.

Ritter, E., and Kinnier Wilson, J. V. 1980. "Prescriptions for an Anxiety State: A Study of *BAM* 234," *Anatolian Studies* 30: 23–30.
Robinson, T. M. 2006. "The Defining Features of Mind–Body Dualism in the Writings of Plato," in *Psyche and Soma*, ed. J. P. Wright and P. Potter (Oxford), 37–55.
Robson, E. 2008. *Mathematics in Ancient Iraq* (Princeton).
Rochberg, F. 2004. *The Heavenly Writing* (Cambridge).
Röllig, W., and Tsukimoto, A. 1999. "Mittelassyrische Texte zum Anbau von Gewürzpflanzen," in *Minuscula Mesopotamica* (Fs. Johannes Renger), ed. B. Böck, E. Cancik-Kirschbaum, and T. Richtera (Münster), 427–43.
Rosenbaum, E. E. 1988. *A Taste of My Own Medicine* (New York).
Russo, L. 2004. *The Forgotten Revolution* (Berlin).
Schnabel, P. 1923. *Berossos und die babylonisch-hellenistische Literatur* (Hildesheim).
Schramm, W. 2008. *Ein Compendium sumerisch-akkadischer Beschwörungen* (Göttingen).
Schuster-Brandis, A. 2008. *Steine als Schutz- und Heilmittel. Untersuchung zu ihrer Verwendung in der Beschwörungskunst Mesopotamiens im 1. Jt. v. Chr.* (Münster).
Schwemer, D. 2007. *Abwehrzauber und Behexung* (Wiesbaden).
Scurlock, J. 1999. "Physician, Exorcist, Conjurer, Magician: A Tale of Two Healing Professionals," in *Mesopotamian Magic: Textual, Historical, and Interpretative Perspectives*, ed. T. Abusch and K. van der Toorn (Groningen), 69–79.
Scurlock, J. 2006. *Magico-Medical Means of Treating Ghost-induced Illnesses in Ancient Mesopotamia* (Leiden).
Shibata, D. 2008. "A Nimrud Manuscript of the Fourth Tablet of the Series *mīs pî*: CTN IV 170 (+) 188 and a *Kiutu* Incantation to the Sun God," *Iraq* 70: 189–204.
Stol, M. 1991–2. "Diagnosis and Therapy in Babylonian Medicine," *JEOL* 32: 42–65.
Stol, M. 1993. *Epilepsy in Babylonia* (Groningen).
Stol, M. 1999. "Psychomatic Suffering in Ancient Mesopotamia," in *Mesopotamian Magic*, ed. T. Abusch and K. van der Toorn (Groningen), 57–68.
Stol, M. 2000. *Birth in Babylonia and the Bible: Its Mediterranean Setting* (Groningen).
Stol, M. 2007. "Fevers in Babylonia," in *Disease in Babylonia*, ed. I. L. Finkel and M. J. Geller (Leiden), 1–39.
Streck, M. 1999. "Hammurabi oder Hammurapi?" *ArOr* 67: 655–69.
Tavernier, J. 2008. "KADP 36: Inventory, Plant List, or Lexical Exercise," *Proceedings of the 51st Rencontre Assyriologique Internationale* (Chicago), 191–202.
Tecusan, M. 2004. *The Fragments of the Methodists*, vol. 1 (Leiden).
Temkin, O. 1956. *Soranus' Gynecology* (Baltimore).
Temkin, O. 1995. *Hippocrates in a World of Pagans and Christians* (Baltimore).

Thureau-Dangin, F. 1922. *Tablettes d'Uruk à l'usage des prêtres du temple d'Anu au temps des Séleucides* (TCL 6), (Paris).

Tsukimoto, A. 1985. *Untersuchungen zur Toten pflege (kispum) im alten Mesopotamien* (Neukirchen-Vluyn).

Ungnad, A. 1944. "Besprechungskunst und Astrologie in Babylonien," *AfO* 14: 251–84.

Unschuld, P. 2003. *Was ist Medizin? Westliche und östliche Wege der Heilkunst* (Munich).

Valance, J. 2000. "Doctors in the Library: The Strange Tale of Apollonius the Bookworm and Other Stories," in *The Library of Alexandria, Centre of Learning in the Ancient World*, ed. R. MacLeod (London), 95–113.

van der Eijk, P. 2000. *Diocles of Carystus* (Leiden).

van der Spek, R. J. 2001. "The Theatre of Babylon in Cuneiform," *Veenhof Anniversary Volume*, ed. W. H. van Soldt, J. G. Dercksen, N. J. C. Kouwenberg, Th. Krispijn (Leiden), 445–56.

van der Toorn, K. 1985. *Sin and Sanction in Israel and Mesopotamia* (Assen).

van Dijk, J. J., and Geller, M. J. 2003. *Ur III Incantations from the Frau Hilprecht Collection, Jena* (Wiesbaden).

van Driel, G. 2002. *Elusive Silver* (Leiden).

Veldhuis, N. 1997. *Elementary Education at Nippur: The Lists of Trees and Wooden Objects* (Groningen).

Villard, P. 1997. "L'éducation d'Assurbanipal," *Ktema* 22: 135–49.

von Staden, H. 1998. *The Art of Medicine in Early Alexandria* (Cambridge).

von Weiher, E. 1983. *Spätbabylonische Texte aus Uruk, Teil II* (Berlin).

von Weiher, E. 1988. *Spätbabylonische Texte aus Uruk, Teil III* (Berlin).

Walker, C. B. F. 1990. "Cuneiform," in *Reading the Past*, J. T. Hooker (London), 15–73.

Watson, G. 1966. *Theriac and Mithridatum: A Study in Therapeutics* (London).

Westbrook, R. 2005. "Patronage in the Ancient Near East," *JESHO* 48: 210–33.

Westenholz, J., and Sigrist, M. 2006. "The Brain, the Marrow, and the Seat of Cognition in Mesopotamian Tradition," *JMC* 7: 1–10.

Wiggermann, F. A. M. 2007. "Some Demons of Time and their Functions in Mesopotamia," in *Die Welt die Götter*, ed. B. Groneberg and H. Spieckermann (Berlin), 102–16.

Wiggermann, F. A. M. 2008. "A Babylonian Scholar in Assur," in *Studies in Ancient Near Eastern World View and Society* (Fs. Stol), ed. R. J. van der Spek (Bethesda), 203–34.

Worthington, M. 2003. "A Discussion of Aspects of the UGU Series," *JMC* 2: 2–13.

Worthington, M. 2005. "Edition of UGU 1 (*BAM* 480 etc.)," *JMC* 5: 6–43.

Worthington, M. 2007. "Addenda and Corrigenda to 'Edition of UGU 1'," *JMC* 9: 43–6.

Wunsch, C. 2007. "The Egibi Family," in G. Leick, *The Babylonian World* (Abingdon), 236–47.

Subject Index

Selective Index of Akkadian and Greek Words

Akkadian Words

abbukatu 155
abriqqu 46
adû 80
agašgû 132
ahhāzu 157
aluzinnu 53
antašubbû 34
apkallu 16, 121
āšipu 43–50, 129, 165
āšipūtu 43–4, 49–50, 76, 111, 162–5
ašqulālu 156
asû 43–4, 46, 49–52, 53, 56, 72, 77, 85, 88, 96, 122, 125–30, 132, 134, 157, 162, 165–7
asûtu 53, 89, 111, 129, 157, 162–5
awīlu 58–60
azallû 156

balītu 157
baluhhu 157
bārû 50–2, 57, 75, 77, 80, 126, 142
bārûtu 50–1, 75–6
bēl nēmeqi 120
bēl šipti 120
bennu 34, 64
bulṭu (*latku*) 64, 82
burallu 85
burāšu 157
būšānu 110

dāgil iṣṣūri 80
dāmu 156
dannatu 143
di'u 151

ērib bīti 50
eṭemmu 155

gallābu 53, 167

hakammu 64
halqu 76
himiṭ ṣēti 63, 151
hunṭu 82–3, 86
huṣṣu 151, 154

ihzu 120, 135, 137
ilku 77
imtu 152
išippu 69

kabābu 151
kalû 75, 77, 137
kalûtu 76

Greek Words

Index of Akkadian Personal Names

Akkadian Divine Names

Printed in the United States
By Bookmasters